Drugs of Abuse

Pharmacology and Molecular Mechanisms

Drugs of Abuse

Pharmacology and Molecular Mechanisms

Sherrel G. Howard, Ph.D.

Molecular and Medical Pharmacology and Child Psychiatry
University of California, Los Angeles

WILEY Blackwell

Library of Congress Cataloging-in-Publication Data

Howard, Sherrel G., author.
  Drugs of abuse : pharmacology and molecular mechanisms / Sherrel G. Howard.
      p. ; cm.
  Includes bibliographical references and index.
  ISBN 978-1-118-28845-0 (cloth)
  I. Title.
  [DNLM: 1. Central Nervous System Agents–metabolism.   2. Street Drugs–pharmacology.
3. Substance-Related Disorders–therapy.   QV 76.5]
  RC564
  362.29–dc23
                                                                    2013045068

Dedication

This book is dedicated to my son, Jon-Erik Akashi and my students in NS 182, from whom I have learned so much.

Contents

Contributor List   ix

Preface   xi

Acknowledgments   xiii

1   Introduction   1

Part I Stimulants   **13**

2   Biochemistry of Neurotransmission   15

3   Amphetamine and Amphetamine Analogs   33

4   Cocaine   65

Part II Depressants, Sedative Hypnotics, and Anxiolytics   **75**

5   Benzodiazepines and Barbiturates   77

Part III Dissociative Anesthetics   **93**

6   Phencyclidine and Ketamine   95

7   γ Hydroxybutyrate   105

Part IV Analgesics   **115**

8   Morphine and Morphine Analogs   117
Carlos Cepeda

Part V Hallucinogens   **135**

9   Lysergic Acid Diethylamide and Mescaline   137

10   Marijuana   153

11   Inhalants and Miscellaneous Drugs   167

Part VI Recovery and Relapse   **181**

12   Treatment of Substance Dependency   183
Mark DeAntonio

Index   189

Contributor List

Carlos Cepeda, Ph.D.
Department of Psychiatry and Pharmacology
University of California, Los Angeles

Mark DeAntonio, M.D.
Department of Child Psychiatry
University of California, Los Angeles

Preface

In Florida, a naked man was found on a bridge chewing the face of another until killed by the police. The man was under the influence of "bath salts", an easy formulation that can be obtained cheaply online. In Canada, pharmacies are robbed at gunpoint to take hold of the last dose of a painkiller withdrawn by the government due to increased recreational use. Date rape drugs are used and abused by teenagers all over the world and emergency rooms at hospitals are at full capacity trying to save the lives of people who have overdosed on ecstasy or heroin.

The need for a book on the pharmacology of addictive drugs has become more critical as the number of people taking drugs around the world continues to rise. While primarily intended for college students, this book was made understandable enough to address the needs of a larger audience, anxious to learn about drugs of abuse. When dealing with potentially addictive drugs, we must leave behind the idea that ignorance is bliss. In our modern society we must realize that ignorance is a risk and knowledge is bliss. Knowing the risks that drugs of abuse generate will hopefully make people think twice before taking a drug.

We have tried to remain neutral when describing the value or dangers of these drugs, neither condemning nor condoning their use. For each one, we have tried to sketch a complete picture of the mechanisms of action, central nervous system (CNS) effects, pharmacokinetics and possible treatment. While making it simple, the scientific aspects of drug effects and mechanisms were not neglected and multiple sources of primary and secondary information were consulted.

We firmly believe that in this book, the reader will find a rich source of important facts and also a glimmer of hope in a world where the drug cartels and unscrupulous governments are attempting to gain control of our children. A more rational use of natural or synthetic, potentially addictive drugs, based on scientific facts is the only way to prepare future generations to face the dangers of abuse and physical dependence.

Acknowledgments

I would like to thank Ms Donna Crandall for all of her work turning my words and ideas into figures. Her creativity and understanding are more than appreciated.

I would also like to thank Dr. Arthur Cho and Dr. James Waschek for their critical reading of parts of the manuscript.

1 Introduction

Learning Objectives

The student will learn:

1. To identify when drug seeking becomes a problem.
2. What is the common link between many dependence-producing drugs?
3. To recognize the common attributes of dependence- producing drugs.
4. Identify the factors involved in drug dependence.

We are a society of drug users. If our headaches or a muscle twinges a little, we take a pill. If we are nervous, "stressed-out," or just cannot sleep, we take a tranquilizer or sleeping pill. If we do not eat a balanced diet, we take vitamin pills, and then diet pills so we can lose the weight we gained because we were not eating a balanced diet. In fact, it almost seems that there is a pill for pretty much everything that is not "just right." As a society we have come to depend on pills, as if the pills would correct any mistakes we make, cure any loneliness or failure we have. However, if we examine societies through the ages, we can see that our society today, is not that different, we just have a wider selection of "cure-alls."

For many thousands of years humans have searched for ways to modify or alter their feeling of well-being and consciousness. We have sought to increase our awareness, decrease boredom, increase alertness, physical prowess, stimulate creativity, or enhance our senses. Throughout the ages we have used potions, plants, extracts, tonics, pills, and injections. All were used to achieve an altered state of consciousness. While there are many ways to achieve this altered state of reality, over the centuries man has chosen to use psychoactive drugs.

Most of the psychoactive drugs consumed were done so by personal choice, rather than professional advice. While society today does not generally approve of this unauthorized use of mind-altering drugs, this has

---

Drugs of Abuse: Pharmacology and Molecular Mechanisms, First Edition. Sherrel G. Howard.
© 2014 John Wiley & Sons, Inc. Published 2014 by John Wiley & Sons, Inc.

not always been the case. Many of the drugs of abuse have had a very colorful history and have often been used not only for their ability to alter perception, but also to gain political, economic, and religious control over a given population.

ORGANIZATION

The first two chapters of this book lay the groundwork or background information for the drugs that will be covered. In this chapter we begin our studies on drug abuse with a brief historical perspective and an introduction to the attitude of society today toward most addictions. We will define the processes that are related to forming an addiction, and define terms that we will be using throughout this book.

Chapter 2 describes the basic steps in the synthesis and metabolism of the neurotransmitters that are primarily involved in producing the effects of a drug. The receptors of these neurotransmitters will also be considered as a potential site to enhance or inhibit drug effects. In Chapters 3–11, the different categories of drugs are examined in regard to their mechanism of action and their clinical and nonclinical usage. The final chapter examines treatment programs and the success and failures of these programs.

The primary focus throughout this book is the mechanisms by which abused drugs exert their effects on both the central and peripheral nervous system. We will examine how tolerance and dependence, both physical and psychological, develop.

OPIUM, MORPHINE, AND HEROIN

Opium has a long and colorful history. Opium is an extract of the opium poppy, and the first recorded use of opium was in Assyria, dating back

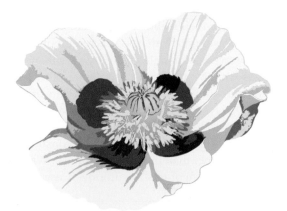

Figure 1.1   Flower of Opium Poppy.

to the seventh century BC. However, records were also found in Samaria, now called Iran, in the year 4000 BC describing the harvest and production of opium. It was harvested and the opium extracted from the poppy seed in much the same way as it is today. The use of opium was also much the same as today, namely, reduction of pain and diarrhea, and the altered mental state of euphoria and sedation was often considered an extra benefit. Because opium was so potent, both the rulers and the holy men used opium to exert control over society.

Opium is referred to in the Iliad, where Helen of Troy mixed a potion of "freedom from grief and pain," and everyone from Hippocrates to Galen described its various uses. During the Dark Ages, around 1000 AD, the use of opium was described in the Arab world. The Arabs then took opium to China in the ninth century and later China imported opium from India. The Chinese initially used opium to treat dysentery. Somewhat later the East India Company imported opium from China, taking it to Portugal. This use was not for the treatment of any disease.

By the seventeenth century opium was a common ingredient in many potions throughout Europe, but there were so many ingredients in these potions that very little harm was caused to the patient because of the opium content. Around the turn of the eighteenth century, the medical profession became concerned with the lavish use of opium. They were largely ignored, as most people saw no great harm coming from its use. In 1800, a German pharmacist isolated a pure alkaloid base from opium and published a paper describing the compound. This paper was completely ignored by the professional community. Twenty years later he published the same paper, only this time he called the substance morphine, the god of sleep and the paper received a lot of attention.

During the seventeenth century, all medicines were taken orally since intravenous injections were very difficult. In 1656 Christopher Wren introduced the hypodermic needle. This was not as much of an improvement as you might think as the needle had a blunt end. To use the hypodermic needle, an incision had to be made in the skin before the needle could be introduced. Surprisingly, it took many years before a bevel was added to the needle, making it possible to insert the needle without cutting the skin first. However, the introduction of the hypodermic needle and syringe added a whole new dimension to the use of opium.

Economics soon became the primary concern in the Opium Wars beginning in Europe. The British were producing opium in India, to sell to the Chinese in exchange for tea. During the American Civil War, opium or a derivative and a hypodermic needle were given to soldiers to alleviate the pain of injuries obtained during battle. Morphine was so widely used that the addiction to morphine was called the "soldier's disease," but was considered preferable to alcohol, as the soldiers were quieter after using morphine. Morphine was now so readily available that it was used to treat any and all painful states.

By the nineteenth century morphine was added to many over-the-counter remedies. It was used to cure alcoholics of their drinking habit and was very popular. McMunn's Elixir of Opium and Mrs. Winslow's Soothing Syrup were the most popular, containing heroin, opium, cocaine, and some alcohol. Mrs. Winslow's Soothing Syrup was used to stop crying, pain from teething, and any small cough that occurred in infants. Children were dying from the overuse of Mrs. Winslow's syrup by young, overprotective mothers.

By the 1900s, opium, heroine, and morphine were so commonly used that a very nice leather pouch could be purchased at Macy's Department Store containing, a vial of heroin, a vial of cocaine, and a reusable hypodermic needle. These kits were well advertised in newspapers and magazines, and at the time, the use of these drugs was well accepted by society.

In 1914, spurred on by the overuse of Mrs. Winslow's Soothing Syrup, the Pure Food and Drug Act and the Harrison Narcotics Act were passed. These two Acts eliminated the over-the-counter sale of narcotics in any form. Of course the passing of these laws made way for the illegal sale of drugs throughout the country.

This brings us to the twentieth century, where drug abuse is no longer accepted by society, and various ways to stop drug abuse where funded by the government, namely, treatment, intervention, and prevention ("just say NO"). Treatment centers sprung up around the country, primarily on the East coast where heroin addiction was being treated with the replacement drug, methadone. The different interventions were an attempt to bring the heroin addict under control. The goal was to protect society from the drug addict, not to produce a drug-free addict.

The Vietnam War saw a new type of addict, who were well educated and well off. When they returned from Vietnam, these addicts quickly overcame their drug "habit"; the demonstrators who remained in the United States were the new and more affluent drug users. This group was more against the direction of our society than the previous drug users, who were escaping pain, disease, or a very hard life. There was a resurgence in heroin use during the 1980s and 1990s and because it was a very lucrative market, Colombian drug lords added heroin to their already lucrative trade in cocaine. Mexican brown and Mexican black tar heroin flooded the market, and as the money increased, other countries, that is, the Golden Triangle in Asia, and Afghanistan also started smuggling heroin into the country. According to the 2003 National Survey on Drug Use and Health, almost four million Americans were using heroin, and the demographics show that new users are younger and coming from more affluent communities. Unfortunately, in 2013, there is again a rise in heroin use among the young educated people in our society.

AMPHETAMINES AND COCAINE

The coca leaf is the natural source of cocaine. It has been in use by the Incas in the Andes Mountains of South America since the eleventh or twelfth century. The coca leaf was controlled by the ruling class and valued far more than gold. Natives used the leaf so they could work in the mountains and not feel pain or tiredness.

During the 1800s cocaine was introduced into Europe. Dr. Sigmund Freud used cocaine on his patients and his good friend Dr. Koller, an ophthalmologist, demonstrated its anesthetic properties and used it in his practice for ophthalmic surgery. An Italian, Mr. Mariani, added coca leaves to red wine, and called it Vin Mariani. It was advertised as a wine to lift one's mood, energy, and spirit. Vin Mariani was thought so highly of that Mr. Mariani received letters of commendation from numerous famous people, one even from the Pope, praising his wine as a gift to humanity.

Cocaine use was more restricted to affluent society because of the cost. However, with the introduction of "crack cocaine" or the free base, it became cheap and easily obtained by anyone. The 1980s were a time when stimulant abuse was increasing and the introduction of a cheap stimulant, that is, crack cocaine, produced a major change in the demographics of the drug culture that could not have been predicted.

Amphetamine, although first synthesized in the late 1800s was not extensively used until World War II. Soldiers on both sides were routinely given amphetamine to fight battle fatigue and increase endurance and outlook. Amphetamine and analogs of amphetamine became popular after the war as a tool to fight weight gain, and are still used for that purpose today. However, a more serious epidemic developed from the use of methamphetamine and methylene-dioxy-methamphetamine (MDMA or Ecstasy).

LYSERGIC ACID DIETHYLAMIDE AND OTHER HALLUCINOGENS

Hallucinogens are drugs that severely distort a person's sense of reality. The psychedelic drugs originally used came from plants, primarily members of the nightshade family or from mushrooms, such as peyote. As early as 1500 BC, tribal medicine men referred to the use of henbane or mandrake root as a means to alleviate pain, act as a poison, or produce hallucinations leading to some type of prophecy.

An additional psychedelic comes from ergot, a naturally occurring purple fungus that comes from mold and grows on rye or wheat. This was quite common during the Middle Ages, and was not uncommon for individual farmers or whole villages to go seemingly mad. An exaggerated

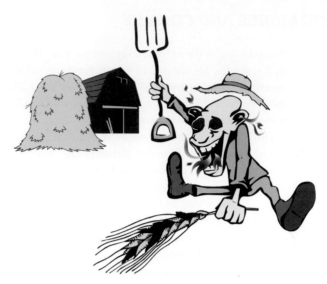

Figure 1.2 An exaggerated cartoon of a farmer during the Middle Ages afflicted with ergot poisoning.

cartoon of a farmer in the Middle Ages afflicted with ergot poisoning can be found in Fig. 1.2. Ergot poisoning does not just produce a "daffy" horse in the field, it occurs most commonly in contaminated grain used for cereal, and is occasionally found even today. This ergot poisoning was given the name "St. Anthony's Fire" and the cure for this "insanity" was to make a pilgrimage to a particular shrine in France. This pilgrimage did in fact cure the affliction, as the mold did not grow in that region of France. The symptoms of this disease are pronounced mental disturbance and a severe vasoconstriction, which is very painful and can lead to gangrene. There has also been speculation that ergot poisoning may have been responsible for the Salem Witch Trials in the seventeenth century; however, there is very little evidence to support this idea.

Ergot mold is the natural form of lysergic acid diethylamide (LSD). Albert Hoffmann was a chemist working for Sandoz Laboratories in Switzerland. In 1943 he synthesized a compound called LSD-25 that he hoped would be an aid to patients with respiratory and/or circulatory problems. In fact LSD-25 is the most potent mood-altering hallucinogen known to man. LSD permeated the culture of the 1960s, from the universities to the music. Hoffmann later wrote about LSD in a book entitled "My Problem Child."

MARIJUANA

The use of cannabis has been recorded for thousands of years. In the year 2737 BC the emperor of China wrote that there were many medicinal uses

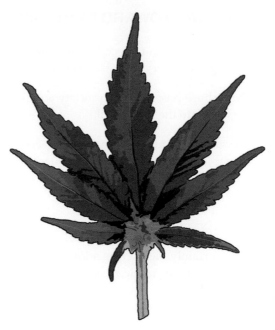

Figure 1.3   Marijuana leaf.

for cannabis, ranging from female disorders to rheumatism. However, in writings from Taoist priests, it is obvious that they were aware of the hallucinogenic properties of Marijuana, and thought it was a useful tool for telling the future.

Marijuana was used in India around 1500 BC as a means to promote good health and also as a means for becoming closer to God. Its use reached Eastern Europe by approximately 500 BC where the burning plant smoke was inhaled in small tents to promote "joy." Most often however, the Marijuana or hemp was most highly prized as a source of fiber, edible seeds, and as a medicine.

Marijuana (hemp) was grown in America in the 1700s by the founding fathers. This was to establish a textile and rope industry in the newly formed country. It is difficult to say whether any of the founding fathers smoked the marijuana leaf, as there is no recorded documentation.

If mind-altering drugs have been around for such a long time and have even enjoyed a certain degree of acceptance by society, why is drug use so frowned upon today? The effects of drug addiction on society and the individual will be discussed briefly in this chapter. We will then cover the transmitters that are involved in drug addiction and the effects of the different drugs on the central and peripheral nervous system. These two chapters provide the groundwork for our studies of abused drugs.

SOCIETY'S ATTITUDE TOWARD DRUG USE

Why is drug use so frowned upon today? The answer is unfortunately very pragmatic. Very often the primary interest is one of cost-benefit.

Drug abuse poses a cost to society and the cost is thought to outweigh the benifit to the individual.

The reasons why a particular drug constitutes a problem to society are complex. The drug and its pharmacological activity are only a starting point. If we consider the three most commonly used nontherapeutic drugs, they are as follows.

Caffeine, Nicotine, and Alcohol

Society certainly views drug addiction very differently from other forms of addiction, for example, *Monday Night Football*, sex, over eating and even coffee, these addictions are not viewed as negatively as drug addiction. Nicotine was once widely accepted; however, it is now viewed very negatively. Alcohol produces a mixed response. It is accepted, in fact, almost expected of one to drink socially; however, if one loses control, then it is viewed very negatively.

The drugs of abuse, both prescription and illegal drugs, form a heterogeneous group pharmacologically. One primary link is that the drug user finds the effect of the drug pleasurable and wants to repeat or sustain the effect or feelings produced by the drug.

This pleasure-seeking effect becomes a problem when the following happens.

1. Drug seeking dominates one's lifestyle.
2. Use of the drug prevents a person from living a lifestyle that society can accept.
3. The desire or craving for the drug begins to dominate the person's life.
4. The "habit" causes actual harm to the individual or community.

One common link of many of the dependence-producing drugs is that of ACTIVATING the mesolimbic dopamine system. When dopamine (DA) receptors are activated, this initiates a complex chain of events in the signal transduction pathway. The common link or response to the various types of psychoactive drugs is that they produce an effect, which we will call rewarding or pleasurable. These same drugs can be tested in the laboratory to determine the effect on an animal's behavior. Animals will self-administer most of the dependence-producing drugs. The effect of the drug is said to have a reinforcing property. This means that whatever behavior the animal was performing at the time the drug was delivered, the probability of its occurring again will increase, thus causing the drug to be administered again. In humans, there is the initial period of drug exposure, or conditioning, before a dependency is formed. The rewarding property of the drug, combined with repeated exposure, usually produces dependence. At this point, taking the drug is now the reward; not being allowed to take the drug is a punishment or a negative reinforcement.

The intensity of the withdrawal syndrome, when the drug is removed, varies depending on the class of drugs. Now drug-seeking behavior is more likely sustained because of the psychological dependence, rather than the severity of the physical withdrawal symptoms.

We should first begin by defining the terms we will be using.

Drug dependence describes the state when drug taking becomes compulsive, taking precedence over other needs.

Drug addiction (an older term) implies a state of physical dependence.

Physical dependence is used to describe the response of the body, when a drug is eliminated. There is a characteristic withdrawal syndrome, suggesting that the person is dependent on the drug.

Psychological dependence refers to a behavioral dependence; this dependence is characterized by a high degree of relapse and continued craving for the drug after termination of use.

Tolerance is a decrease in the pharmacological effect of a drug, upon repeated administration of the drug. Thus, it will take a greater amount of the drug to produce the same effect.

A common feature of these various types of drugs (psychoactive drugs) is that they produce dependence. Dependence is produced primarily because there is a rewarding or positive effect from the drug.

Dependence

The term positive reinforcement is used to define the repeated occurrence of a response after administration of a drug. If after repeated administration of a drug, the drug is removed or no longer administered, then removal of the drug constitutes a negative reinforcement.

The physical withdrawal syndrome, which is associated with the state of physical dependence, is one manifestation of addiction. The intensity of the physical withdrawal symptoms varies and is particularly pronounced in the case of opioid withdrawal.

Lastly, conditioning also plays a role in sustaining drug dependence.

If we consider heroin or nicotine, in the case of these drugs, environment plays an important role. The sight of the syringe or a cigarette, a smell, a coffee shop, or even a particular person, anything can become associated with the pleasurable experience of the drug, such that the stimulus (i.e. the cigarette, person or place etc.) evokes the response or craving. This was demonstrated many years ago in the experiment Pavlov performed using a conditioned stimulus, that is, a bell. When a hungry dog smelled food, it began to salivate. If a bell was rung every time the dog was fed, the bell soon became associated with food. Finally, the sound of the bell alone produced salivation.

Reward Pathways

An important reward pathway involved in the formation of drug dependence is the mesolimbic dopaminergic pathway. DA coming from the ventral midbrain (A10 cell group) projects to the nucleus accumbens and limbic region. This pathway constitutes a reward pathway.

All of the drugs that we will discuss produce dependence. This includes the opioids, marijuana, amphetamines, and cocaine. All of these drugs produce an INCREASE in the release of DA. This initiates a complex chain of events in the signal transduction pathway for the neurotransmitter DA. Chronic treatment with drugs like opioids or cocaine increases the amount of adenylate cyclase and other components in the signaling pathway including G proteins. Increases in cAMP, produces changes in cell function through a cAMP-dependent protein kinase, which controls ion channels.

Summary

The factors involved in drug dependence:

1. The psychoactive drugs produce an effect that is pleasurable and could be defined as a reward.
2. Continued use produces a dependency such that withdrawal of the drug produces a physical withdrawal syndrome.
3. The psychological dependence can last far longer than the physical dependence.

To summarize the important facts:

1. Dependence develops after multiple uses of a psychoactive drug.
2. The psychoactive drugs that produce dependence are varied and act through a variety of different neurochemical mechanisms.
3. The common attribute of all of these dependence-producing drugs is that they produce a feeling of euphoria or act as a "reward" which makes one feel good.

Common attributes of dependence-producing drugs:

1. A tolerance develops.
2. The withdrawal syndrome occurs, to a greater or lesser degree, if the drug is removed.

3. A strong psychological dependence is also formed, which is associated with subtle cues or stimuli.
4. The psychological dependence is long lasting and can lead to relapse.

Review Questions

1. Is there a relationship between physical dependence and tolerance?
2. How does a drug act as a positive reinforcer?
3. Why does society view addiction so negatively?

REFERENCES AND ADDITIONAL READING

Ashton CH. 2001. Pharmacology and effects of cannabis: a brief review. *Br. J. Psychiatry.* 178:101–106.

Buttner A. 2011. Review: The neuropathology of drug abuse. *Neuropathol. Appl. Neurobiol.* 37:118–134.

Kalivas PW. and Volkow ND. 2005. The neural basis of addiction: a pathology of motivation and choice. *Am. J. Psychiatry.* 162:1403–1413.

Khantzian EJ. 1985. The self-medication hypothesis of addictive disorders: focus on heroin and cocaine dependence. *Am. J. Psychiatry.* 142:1259–1264.

Part I   Stimulants

2 Biochemistry of Neurotransmission

Learning Objectives

The student will be able to:

1. Describe the synthesis and metabolism of transmitters involved in abused drugs.
2. Outline the process from synthesis to storage of a neurotransmitter.
3. Know at least two ways that a drug could interfere with neurotransmission.
4. Explain the role of glutamate in the release of dopamine (DA).
5. Identify the enzymes and cofactors involved in the synthesis of the catechol and indolamines.

ADRENERGIC TRANSMISSION

An understanding of the adrenergic neuron is important both as a target of drug action and as a site for clinically useful drugs. Over the last 100 years our knowledge of drugs and their mechanisms of action as well as the biochemistry of the nerve ending have made enormous leaps forward. In this chapter we will review the basic biochemistry of the various neurotransmitters that are involved with the physiological actions that are seen with the drugs we are studying.

HISTORICAL OVERVIEW

In 1913, Sir Henry Dale demonstrated that adrenaline (epinephrine) produced both vasoconstriction and vasodilatation. However, it was not until 1946 that von Euler demonstrated that it was norepinephrine (NE) that

---

Drugs of Abuse: Pharmacology and Molecular Mechanisms, First Edition. Sherrel G. Howard.
© 2014 John Wiley & Sons, Inc. Published 2014 by John Wiley & Sons, Inc.

was the transmitter in the mammalian peripheral sympathetic neuron and not epinephrine. Over the following 10 years, NE was conclusively identified as a neurotransmitter. Shortly thereafter, experiments demonstrated that NE was released from the neuron terminal in the peripheral nervous system and it was also found in brain tissue. It was not until the development of the fluorescent histochemical method, which made it possible to visualize catecholamines, that the morphology of the peripheral neuron and the distribution of catecholamines in the brain could be determined.

The development of the Falck–Hillarp fluorescent histochemical method was a major scientific advance, making it possible to visualize the neuron terminal and the axon varicosities of three neurotransmitter systems, dopamine (DA), NE, and serotonin (5-hydroxytryptamine, 5-HT). Fluorescent histochemistry can, in part, be credited with the finding that DA was more than a precursor of NE, but was also a neurotransmitter. During the late 1960s numerous studies came out of Sweden from members of the "Catecholamine Club" examining the role of DA and 5-HT in the brain.

During the last half of the twentieth century, numerous studies were performed to identify the means by which the catecholamines were synthesized, released, and metabolized in the brain and sympathetic neuron. While Blasko, in 1939, hypothesized the enzymatic steps necessary to form NE from the amino acid tyrosine, it was not until 1964 that Nagatsu and coworkers confirmed experimentally that L-tyrosine was converted to L-DOPA.

BIOSYNTHESIS OF DOPAMINE AND NOREPINEPHRINE

Tyrosine Hydroxylase

Tyrosine hydroxylase is the first enzyme in the biosynthetic pathway of DA and NE (Figure 2.1). Tyrosine hydroxylase oxidizes L-tyrosine to form dihydroxy-phenylalanine. Tyrosine is present in the circulation. It is taken up into nerve endings or chromaffin cells, where it is converted to DA, NE, or epinephrine (Figure 2.1). Only a small part of the available tyrosine is used in the synthesis of neurotransmitter, the rest of the circulating tyrosine is used in the formation of other compounds in the body.

Tyrosine hydroxylase is the rate-limiting step in the synthesis of DA and NE. The enzyme, while not totally selective, demonstrates a high degree of substrate specificity. Tyrosine hydroxylase requires several cofactors.

Specific cofactors required by tyrosine hydroxylase are as follows.

1. Molecular O_2
2. Fe + +
3. Tetrahydropteridine

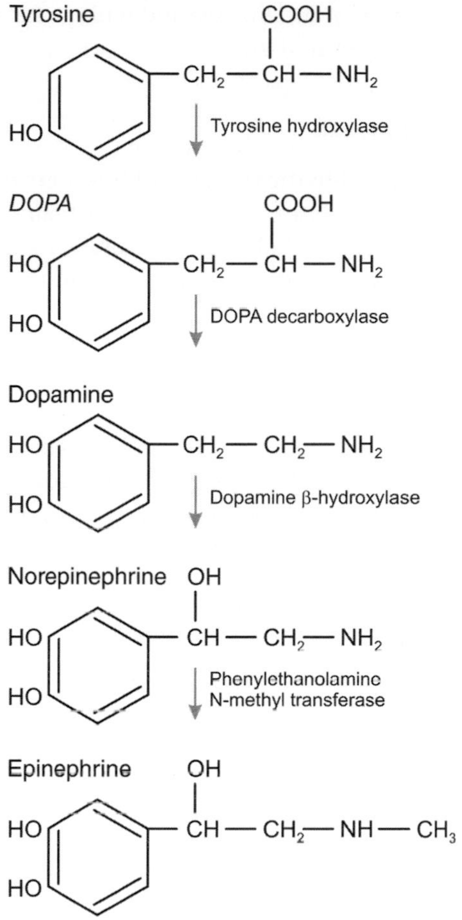

Figure 2.1 Synthetic pathway starting with the precursor L-tyrosine to form DA and norepinephrine.

Inhibition of tyrosine hydroxylase is one effective way to decrease the concentration of DA or NE in the brain or NE in peripheral sympathetically innervated nerves. Additionally, amino acid analogs or catechol derivatives will also inhibit tyrosine hydroxylase.

Dihydroxyphenylalanine Decarboxylase

Dihydroxyphenylalanine (DOPA) decarboxylase does not demonstrate a high degree of specificity and will act on many L-aromatic amino acids. It is somewhat ubiquitous and can be found in many tissues outside of the central nervous system (CNS). DOPA decarboxylase is a very active enzyme with an apparent K_m of 4×10^{-4} M. It requires pyridoxal phosphate (vitamin B_6) as a cofactor. However, unlike tyrosine hydroxylase, reducing the concentration of the cofactor does not significantly decrease the activity of the enzyme and will not result in a decrease in the concentration of DA in tissue.

Dopamine-β-Hydroxylase

Dopamine-β-hydroxylase (DBH) is a mixed function oxidase (as is tyrosine hydroxylase) and is localized mainly in the membrane of storage granules of catecholamine-containing neurons.

Requirements for DBH are as follows.

1.   Molecular O_2
2.   Ascorbic acid

While not a requirement, dicarboxylic acids will stimulate the reaction of converting DA to NE. DBH is a relatively non-specific enzyme and will oxidize most phenylethylamines, occasionally producing compounds that will act as "false transmitters" at the NE nerve ending.

Phenylethanolamine-N-methyltransferase

NE is N-methylated by the enzyme phenylethanolamine-N-methyltransferase to form epinephrine. This occurs primarily in the adrenal medulla, with only very low activity seen in the mammalian brain.

REGULATION OF SYNTHESIS

The most effective way to modulate or alter DA synthesis within the DA neuron would necessarily involve tyrosine hydroxylase, as this is the rate-limiting step in the synthetic pathway.

There are several ways that DA synthesis can be altered which are as follows.

1.   By increasing the concentration of DA, it produces end-product inhibition of tyrosine hydroxylase, which in turn will compete with the biopterin cofactor.
2.   The availability of cofactors, particularly tetrahydrobiopterin may play a role in regulating tyrosine hydroxylase.
3.   Pre-synaptic DA receptors are activated by DA released from the nerve terminal. The concentration of released DA results in a feedback inhibition of DA synthesis. (Evidence suggests that neurotransmitters can regulate their own release by acting on pre-synaptic receptors. This type of regulation by neurotransmitters has been termed "auto-inhibitory feedback mechanism".)

4. Impulse flow is yet another way to regulate DA synthesis. As impulse flow increases, tyrosine hydroxylation is increased. Additionally, when impulse flow increases, tyrosine hydroxylation is regulated by the availability of tyrosine (see point number 1).

RELEASE OF DOPAMINE AND REGULATION OF RELEASE

The release of DA or NE from the nerve terminal occurs when an action potential travels down the axon toward the nerve terminal. Depolarization of the nerve terminal may also occur if the extracellular potassium concentration is increased. The increase in potassium opens calcium channels causing vesicles to fuse with the cell membrane and release the neurotransmitter. This process is called exocytosis (Figure 2.2).

Release of a neurotransmitter can also be modulated by the neurotransmitter itself. DA or NE, acting at their pre-synaptic receptors can stimulate or inhibit the release of the transmitter. Additionally, agonists or antagonists of the neurotransmitters can also stimulate or inhibit the pre-synaptic receptor producing a marked effect on neurotransmission.

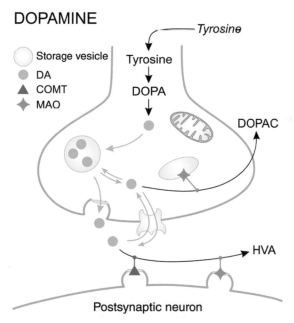

Figure 2.2 Schematic diagram of the dopamine synapse demonstrating the uptake of tyrosine and its conversion to dopamine (DA) in the presynaptic terminal. DA is taken up into vesicles by an active transport mechanism. DA, when released can interact with the post synaptic receptor and/or the presynaptic receptor. The action of DA is terminated by reuptake into the presynaptic terminal by Uptake I. DA is metabolized by MAO or COMT.

Dopamine Uptake

The DA nerve ending possesses high-affinity DA uptake sites. The uptake sites are important in terminating the action of the neurotransmitter. Uptake of the neurotransmitter employs a membrane carrier called the DA transporter (DAT), which transports DA into and out of the nerve ending, depending on the concentration gradient. DA is taken up rapidly after it has been released.

In the mid 1970s, Iversen defined two uptake systems, Uptake I and Uptake II. Uptake I is a high-affinity system with a low maximum rate of uptake. (The role of Uptake I in the mechanism of action of several CNS stimulants will be examined in subsequent chapters). This relatively rapid reuptake of DA not only modulates the concentration of DA in the synapse, but also the amount of time it has to interact with the pre- and post-synaptic receptors.

Storage

Most of the monoamines (DA, NE, and 5-HT) within the nerve terminal are stored in vesicles (Figure 2.2). It requires an active transport mechanism to carry DA through the vesicular membrane. Since this is an active transport mechanism, ATP is required. There are known drugs that can interfere with the storage and transport process, such as reserpine. Reserpine acts by depleting the vesicles of the stores of DA, NE, and 5-HT.

Metabolism

The catecholamines, DA, and NE are metabolized primarily by two enzymes, monoamine oxidase (MAO) and catechol-O-methyltransferase (COMT). After release, DA is taken up into the nerve terminal by the Uptake I carrier. It is converted by intraneuronal MAO to dihydroxyphenylacetic acid (DOPAC) (Figure 2.2).

In most neurons, information is transmitted chemically by the neurotransmitter. The basic steps in the synthesis and release of a neurotransmitter are essentially the same for both the catecholamines (DA and NE) and the indolamines (5-HT). The steps for the primary events following an action potential are illustrated in Figure 2.3. At any of these steps from synthesis to release and reuptake, the effects of a neurotransmitter can be altered or modulated by a drug interaction.

DOPAMINE RECEPTORS

While there are many points in the synthesis and metabolism of a neurotransmitter that can be interrupted or modulated by a drug, receptor-mediated mechanisms provide an important area for drug-receptor interaction.

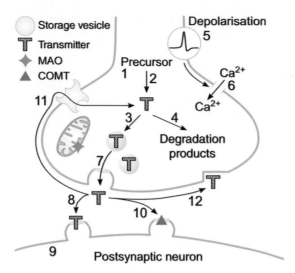

Basic processes at chemically transmitting synapse are as follows.

1. Precursor uptake
2. Transmitter synthesis
3. Transmitter storage in vesicles
4. Surplus transmitter degradation
5. Propagated action potential depolarisation
6. Ca^{2+} influx response to depolarisation
7. Transmitter release by exocytosis
8. Postsynaptic membrane diffusion
9. Postsynaptic receptor interactions
10. Transmitter inactivation
11. Transmitter re-uptake or degradation products
12. Presynaptic receptor interactions

Figure 2.3   Basic Steps in Neurochemical Transmission.

Receptor Subtypes

DA receptors were first characterized as being either a D_1 or a D_2 type of DA receptor. The D_1 and D_2 receptors differ in that they utilize different transduction mechanisms, they have a different distribution in the brain, and they interact differently with adenylate cyclase. DNA cloning has demonstrated that they belong to a large family of G protein-coupled receptors and the two receptors are composed of several novel sub-types.

The D_1 receptor family has one additional subtype, namely the D_5 receptor. The D_5 receptor is pharmacologically similar to the D_1 receptor; however, it has a higher affinity for DA. The D_1 and the D_5 receptors both stimulate adenylate cyclase activity.

The D_2 receptor consists of four subtypes. There are two forms of the D_2 receptor, $D_{2\,short}$ and $D_{2\,long}$. These were identified by gene cloning studies. The two subtypes have identical pharmacology. The third subtype of the D_2 receptor is the D_3 receptor. The D_3 receptor gene has a different

Table 2.1   Potential Sites for Modulating Dopaminergic Function

Site	Effect
Stimulate postsynaptic receptors	Increase transmission of dopamine Increase function of neuronal feedback loops
Block postsynaptic dopamine receptors	Decrease dopamine transmission Interfere with function of neuronal feedback loops
Stimulate presynaptic dopamine autoreceptor	Decrease dopamine synthesis and release Decrease firing rate, decrease output
Block presynaptic dopamine autoreceptors	Increase dopamine synthesis and release

Source: Modified from Cooper et al. (2003).

anatomical distribution and some novel pharmacological characteristics. The fourth subtype is the D_4 receptor gene. It has a high degree of homology with the D_2 and D_3 receptor genes and the pharmacological profile of the D_4 receptor is also similar to that of the D_2 and D_3 receptor subtypes.

To better understand how any given drug will affect both the brain and the behavior of any animal, it is necessary to look at the potential sites of drug action. We have examined the potential sites for drug action (Figure 2.3) within the neuron, that can alter or modulate the function of the DA neuron. Drugs can also have an effect at the various DA receptors to alter or modulate the activity of the neuron, or to alter other transmitter systems, and any of these actions in turn will alter or modulate the functioning of the DA neuron. Consider the potential effects that any DA agonist or antagonist would produce when acting at the DA receptors see Table 2.1.

SEROTONIN (5-HYDROXYTRYPTAMINE)

Since the mid-nineteenth century it was recognized that a substance in serum produced a strong contraction of smooth muscle organs (Aghajanian and Sanders-Bush, 2002). It was not until 1948 that scientists at the Cleveland Clinic identified the substance in clotted blood and called it 5-HT (compare Figure 2.1 and Figure 2.4). Since that time, it has been identified not only in the gastrointestinal tract in high concentrations, but also in the central nervous system.

The biosynthesis and metabolism of 5-HT closely parallels that of DA or NE (Figure 2.1 for comparison).

The precursor for 5-HT is the amino acid tryptophan. Tryptophan is converted to 5-hydroxytryptophan by tryptophan hydroxylase. This first step in the 5-HT synthesis pathway is a rate-limiting step, similar to the synthetic pathway for DA, where tyrosine hydroxylase is the rate-limiting step.

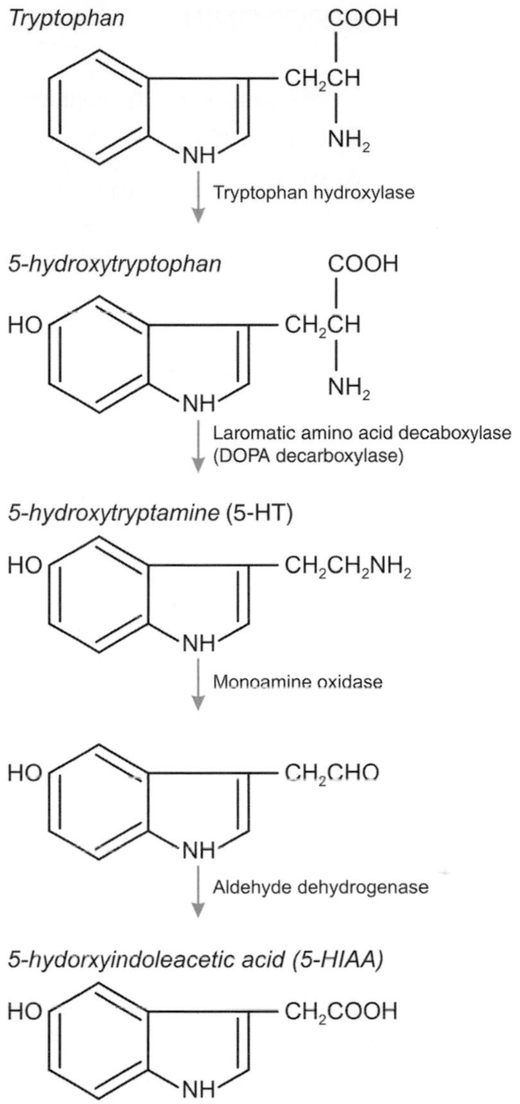

Tryptophan

5-hydroxytryptophan

Tryptophan hydroxylase

5-hydroxytryptamine (5-HT)

*Laromatic amino acid decaboxylase
(DOPA decarboxylase)*

Monoamine oxidase

Aldehyde dehydrogenase

5-hydorxyindoleacetic acid (5-HIAA)

Figure 2.4 The biosynthesis and metabolism of serotonin (5-HT).

Tryptophan hydroxylase requires the following.

1. Molecular oxygen
2. Tetrahydrobiopterin

Synthesis occurs in both neurons and chromaffin cells. 5-hydroxytryptophan is decarboxylated by L-aromatic amino acid decarboxylase, to form 5-hydroxytryptamine. This is the same nonspecific enzyme that was found to decarboxylase DOPA (Figure 2.1).

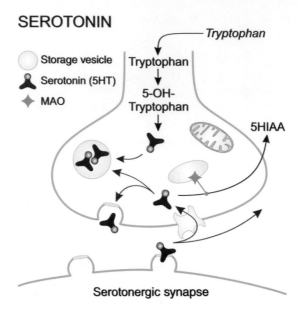

SEROTONIN

- ○ Storage vesicle
- ⚏ Serotonin (5HT)
- ◆ MAO

Tryptophan

Tryptophan
↓
5-OH-
Tryptophan
↓

5HIAA

Serotonergic synapse

Figure 2.5   Schematic diagram of the serotonergic neuron. The diagram illustrates the mechanisms of synthesis, storage release and reuptake.

1. Synthesis. Tryptophan is taken up into the neuron and converted to 5-HT through a series of enzymatic reactions.
2. Storage. 5-HT is transported into the storage vesicles.
3. Release. 5-HT is released from the nerve ending by depolarization.
4. Interaction at the receptor. 5-HT interacts with the pre or postsynaptic receptor.
5. Reuptake. The action of 5-HT is terminated by reuptake into the presynaptic terminal.
6. Metabolism. 5-HT will be metabolized by MAO if it is in a free state within the presynaptic terminal.

There is a high-affinity uptake system for 5-HT that rapidly removes 5-HT from the synaptic cleft, which is similar to that discussed for the catecholamines. If 5-HT is not rapidly taken up into the vesicle for storage it will be metabolized by MAO within the neuron (Figure 2.5). There is also a high affinity uptake system for the uptake of 5-HT into platelets, which occurs in the intestines. The mechanisms by which 5-HT is synthesized, stored, released, and returned to the neuron are very similar to those discussed for catecholamines (compare Figures 2.2 and 2.5).

Metabolism of Serotonin

The most common metabolic pathway of 5-HT is by MAO. The end product, 5-hydroxyindolacetic acid (5-HIAA) is formed after deamination of 5-HT by MAO and further oxidation to 5-HIAA. 5-HT can be metabolized to other end products depending on the ratio of NAD + /NADH.

SEROTONIN RECEPTORS

It has been nearly 50 years since Gaddum and Picarelli first defined the pharmacological properties of 5-HT receptors. At this time they recognized two receptors. Presently there are at least seven families of 5-HT receptor subtypes (and possibly eight). Six 5-HT receptor subtypes are G protein-coupled receptors and one, the $5HT_3$ receptor, is a ligand-gated ion channel receptor. With such diversity, it should not be surprising that the actions of stimulating 5-HT receptors are so complex. Some of the major effects of 5-HT on various systems in the body are listed below.

1. Nerve Endings
   By stimulating the $5HT_3$ receptor, pain mediating, sensory nerve endings are stimulated.
2. Central Nervous System
   5-HT acts at both pre- and post-synaptic nerve endings to excite or inhibit transmitter release. 5-HT in the CNS is involved in modulation of mood, sleep, appetite, temperature regulation, perception of pain, regulation of blood pressure, and vomiting. It is also involved in migraine headaches and depression.
3. Blood Vessels
   5-HT produces constriction in large vessels. This is a direct effect on smooth muscle and is mediated by the 5-HT_{2A} receptor.
   5-HT will produce vasodilation through 5-HT_1 receptors, either by enhancing the release of nitrous oxide (NO) or by inhibiting the release of NE.
4. Platelets
   5-HT increases platelet aggregation.
5. Gastrointestinal tract
   5-HT has a direct effect on smooth muscle cells, so that it will increase GI motility and contraction. This is only a minor effect in humans, although it has a significant effect on other animals.

In Table 2.2 the 5-HT receptors are shown along with their effect on the specific transduction pathways.

The 5-HT receptors are linked to an enormous array of drug actions and clinical conditions. This could only be accomplished with the diversity of receptors and transduction pathways that are found in the serotonergic system (For further reading see suggested readings below).

Summary

1. There are three structures that have high concentrations of 5-HT which are as follows.

(a) Chromafin cells in the gastrointestinal tract.
(b) Platelets.
(c) The central nervous system.
2. The synthesis and metabolism of 5-HT closely parallels the synthesis and metabolism of DA and NE.
3. Tryptophan is the precursor of 5-HT and is obtained from one's diet.
4. 5-HT is taken up or transported into 5-HT-containing neurons by a specific transporter system.
5. Catabolism/degradation occurs primarily by MAO forming 5-HIAA, which is excreted in urine.

Table 2.2   Serotonin Receptor Subtypes and Distribution

Receptor Subtype	Distribution	Post-Receptor Mechanisms
5-HT$_{1A}$	Raphe nuclei hippocampus	Multiple mechanisms G$_i$ coupling dominates
5-HT$_{1B}$	Substantia nigra, globus pallidus, basal ganglia	G$_i$, decrease cAMP
5-HT$_{1Dab}$	Brain	G$_i$, decrease cAMP
5-HT$_{1E}$	Cortex, putamen	G$_i$, decrease cAMP
5-HT$_{1F}$	Cortex, hippocampus	G$_i$, decrease cAMP
5-HT$_{1P}$	Enteric nervous system	G$_o$, slow EPSP
5-HT$_{2A}$	Platelets, smooth muscle, cerebral cortex, skeletal muscle	G$_q$, increase IP3
5-HT$_{2B}$	Stomach fundus	G$_q$, increase IP3
5-HT$_{2C}$	Choroid, hippocampus, substantia nigra	G$_q$, increase IP3
5-HT$_3$	Area postrema, sensory, and enteric nerves	Receptor is Na + -K + ion channel
5-HT$_4$	CNS, myenteric neurons, smooth muscle	G$_s$, increase cAMP
5-HT$_{5A,B}$	Brain	Decrease cAMP
5-HT$_{6,7}$	Brain	G$_s$, increase cAMP

Source: Modified from Katzung et al. (2004).

AMINO ACID NEUROTRANSMITTERS

γ-Aminobutyric Acid

Amino acid neurotransmitters make up the greatest percentage of transmitters in the brain; however, the pharmacology and function of DA, NE, and acetylcholine are better understood. γ-aminobutyric acid (GABA) is an inhibitory neurotransmitter. It is primarily released from interneurons throughout the CNS and spinal cord. GABA is one of the inhibitory amino acid neurotransmitters, while glutamate is one of the excitatory amino acid neurotransmitters.

Synthesis of γ-aminobutyric Acid

Glutamic acid decarboxylase converts L-glutamic acid to GABA. This is a relatively specific decarboxylase, unlike the decarboxylase used in the synthesis of catecholamines. Glutamic acid decarboxylase requires pyridoxal phosphate as a coenzyme.

Storage

GABA is stored in vesicles within the neuron and is transported into the vesicles by a specific GABA transporter. The GABA transporter will also transport other inhibitory neurotransmitters, such as glycine. Glia are also capable of storing GABA. This ability to be stored in glia distinguishes GABA from other neurotransmitters.

Release

When an action potential depolarizes the neuron, GABA is released. GABA can be taken up and thereby inactivated by both neurons and glia. Reuptake, just as with the catecholamines, is the primary means of inactivation and removal from the synaptic cleft (Figure 2.6).

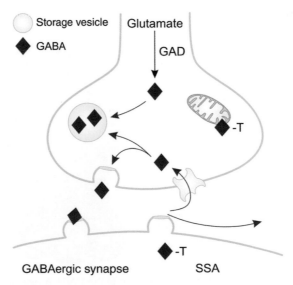

Figure 2.6 Schematic of a GABAergic neuron.

GABA RECEPTORS

GABA_A Receptor

There are two main subtypes of GABA receptors, $GABA_A$ and $GABA_B$. $GABA_A$ receptors are the primary inhibitory transmitter receptor in the CNS and they are the more abundant of the two receptors. The $GABA_A$ receptor can be modulated by benzodiazepines and barbiturates (see Chapter 5). $GABA_A$ is an ionotropic receptor and it is selectively permeable to chloride (Figure 2.7).

GABA_B Receptor

The $GABA_B$ receptor is a member of the G protein-coupled receptors. It is classified as a metabotropic receptor. Unlike the $GABA_A$ receptor, the $GABA_B$ receptor is not linked to a chloride channel and it is not modulated by either barbiturates or benzodiazepines.

A fundamental role for the $GABA_B$ receptor has emerged as being a mediator of slow inhibitory post-synaptic potentials. Activation of the $GABA_B$ receptor also inhibits the release of many of the biogenic amines, as well as GABA through an interaction at the autoreceptor. In contrast to $GABA_A$ receptors, $GABA_B$ receptors are coupled to Ca^{++} or K^+ channels via a second messenger system.

$GABA_B$ receptors are found in both pre- and post-synaptic membranes. They decrease Ca^{++} conductance, facilitate the opening of K^+ channels, and inhibit adenylyl cyclase. The $GABA_B$ receptors are thought to be

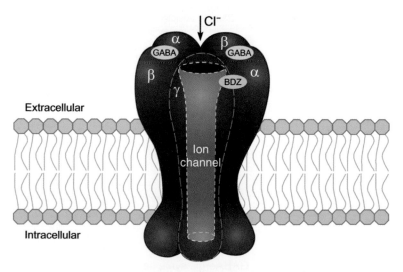

Figure 2.7 Schematic diagram of the GABA A receptor-chloride ion channel macro-molecular complex.

linked to a Ca^{++} channel, possibly through GTP and are only activated under certain physiological conditions.

GLUTAMIC ACID

Glutamic acid is an excitatory amino acid. It was difficult to establish that glutamic acid (GLU) was a neurotransmitter, even though the distribution in the mammalian brain was uneven, with high concentrations only in specific areas. Additionally, GLU produces a powerful stimulatory effect when applied locally to neural tissue. In spite of these data, the status of GLU as a neurotransmitter remained uncertain for many years. GLU did not meet the criteria for being a neurotransmitter in the opinion of many scientists, and it was pointed out that GLU was a precursor in the synthesis of GABA, as well as being involved in the intermediate metabolism of some proteins.

Synthesis of Glutamic Acid

GLU is synthesized from two sources;

a.   transamination of a-oxoglutarate
b.   glutamine

Glutamine is synthesized in glial cells and then transported into nerve terminals where it is acted on by glutaminase to form GLU. GLU synthesis is regulated by end-product inhibition and the newly synthesized GLU is preferentially stored in vesicles and released by exocytosis (which is Ca^{++} dependent) after a nerve impulse depolarizes the nerve terminal (Figure 2.8).

Much like previous transmitters, the action of GLU is terminated primarily by reuptake. GLU is taken up either by a GLU transporter on the neuron that released GLU, or by the GLU transporters on adjacent neurons, by glial cells, or possibly by all three mechanisms.

EXCITATORY AMINO ACID RECEPTORS

Over the past twenty years, advances in technology have made it possible to characterize and isolate many amino acid receptors. Prior to this time, excitatory amino acid receptors were divided into two subtypes, N-methyl-D-aspartate (NMDA) receptors or non-NMDA receptors.

Most neurons are excited by GLU and this activation of GLU receptors includes both the ionotropic and the metabotropic receptors.

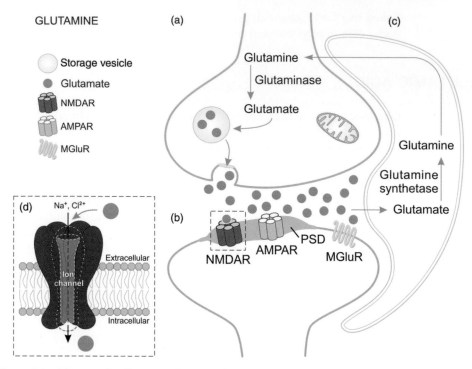

Figure 2.8 Diagram of a Glutamate Synapse. Glutamine is taken up into the glutamatergic neuron (a) The synthesis of glutamate from glutamine by the enzyme glutaminase occurs in the glutamatergic neuron. Glutamate is then taken up into the vesicles by the vesicular glutamate transporter. When released by an action potential, glutamate can interact with AMPA and NMDA ionotropic receptors (AMPAR, NMDAR) on the postsynaptic density (PSD) as well as metabotropic receptors (MGluR) on the postsynaptic cell (b). Neurotransmitter action is terminated by active transport of glutamate into glial cells (c) or by the glutamate transporter. It is converted into glutamine by, glutamine synthetase and exported into the glutamatergic axon. The insert (d) depicts a model NMDA receptor channel complex that consists of a tetrameric protein that is permeable to Na+ and Ca+2 after binding to glutamate. Adapted from Katzung et al. 2009.

The ionotropic receptors consist of three different subtypes based on cloning studies: the a-amino-3-hydroxy-5-methylisoxazole-4-propionic acid (AMPA), kainic acid (KA), and NMDA receptors (Figure 2.8).

AMPA receptors are numerous and found on all neurons. The majority of AMPA receptors are permeable to Na^+ and K^+, but not Ca^{2+}. When AMPA receptors are found on inhibitory interneurons, they tend to be permeable to Ca^{+2}.

Kainate receptors are found in high levels in the hippocampus, cerebellum, and spinal cord. KA receptors are permeable to Na^+ and K^+ and under some conditions to Ca^{2+}.

The NMDA receptor is similar to the AMPA receptor in that it is found on most neurons in the CNS. Unlike the KA and AMPA receptors, NMDA receptors are permeable to all three: Na^+, K^+, and Ca^{2+}.

DOPAMINE AND GLUTAMIC ACID INTERACTION OR "THE GLUTAMATE STORY"

The studies describing the interaction between DA and glutamate have greatly enhanced our knowledge of the mechanism of action of many of the CNS stimulants and helped to explain the diverse behavioral patterns that are found with many of the abused drugs. The focus of this research may also aid in the underlying cause and treatment of schizophrenia, as well as provide alternative treatments for some abused drugs (Bunney et al. 2000).

DA and NMDA receptors have been shown to interact in striatal medium-sized spiny neurons. It has been demonstrated that a variety of responses can be produced by this interaction, and it depends primarily on which DA receptor subtype it is activated (Cepeda and Levine, 1998). If the DA D_1 receptor is activated, the NMDA-mediated response will be enhanced and there will be an increase in GLU released (Kalivas and Duffy, 1995, Figure 2.9). However, in contrast to the DA D_1 effects, if the DA D_2 receptor is activated, there will be a decrease in the NMDA response and a decrease in GLU released (Figure 2.8, Cepeda et al., 1998). Additionally, if the presynaptic DA D_2 receptor is stimulated, there will also be an attenuation of the NMDA response and decrease in GLU released (Figure 2.9).

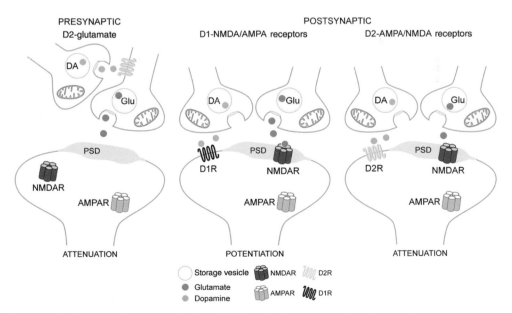

Figure 2.9   The interaction of DA with Glu, NMDA or AMPA receptors. Note the net effect varies depending on which DA receptor is stimulated and whether it is a pre-or post synaptic receptor.

> ## Review Questions
>
> 1. Describe the process of synthesis and storage of the three catechol and indolamines.
> 2. Explain the effect of glutamine release on the release of DA.
> 3. Outline the synthetic pathway for the synthesis of DA and include the enzymes and cofactors. What is the rate-limiting step in this pathway?
> 4. Describe the interaction between DA and NMDA receptors.

REFERENCES AND ADDITIONAL READING

Aghajanian GK, Sanders-Bush E. 2002. Serotonin. In: Davis KL, Charney D, Coyle JT, Nemeroff C (eds), *Neuropsychopharmacology: The Fifth Generation of Progress*. Lippincott Williams & Wilkins, Philadelphia.

Bunney BG, Bunney WE Jr., Carlsson A. 2000. Schizophrenia and glutamate: an update. In: Davis KL, Charney D, Coyle JT, Nemeroff C (eds), *Neuropsychopharmacology: The Fifth Generation of Progress*. Lippincott Williams & Wilkins, Philadelphia.

Cepeda C, Levine MS. 1998. Dopamine and N-methyl-D-aspartate receptor interactions in the neostriatum. *Dev. Neurosci.* 20:1–18.

Cepeda C, Colwell CS, Itri JN, Chandler SH, Levine MS. 1998. Dopaminergic modulation of NMDA-induced whole cell currents in neostriatal neurons in slices: contribution of calcium conductances. *J. Neurophysiol.* 79:82–94.

Cooper JR, Bloom FE, Roth RH. 2003. *The Biochemical Basis of Neuropharmacology*, 8th edn. Oxford University Press.

Kalivas PW, Duffy P. 1995. D1 receptors modulate glutamate transmission in the ventral tegmental area. *J. Neurosci.* 15:5379–5388.

Katzung BG, Masters SB, Trevor AJ. 2004. *Basic and Clinical Pharmacology*, 9th edn. Lange Medical Books/McGraw Hill.

Katzung BG, Masters SB, Trevor AJ. 2009. *Basic and Clinical Pharmacology*, 9th edn. Lange Medical Books/McGraw Hill.

3 Amphetamine and Amphetamine Analogs

Learning Objectives

The student will learn:

1. The meaning of terms such as, indirectly acting sympathomimetic, reuptake, and sympathetic nervous system.
2. The mechanism of action of amphetamine, methamphetamine, and methylenedioxymethamphetamine (MDMA).
3. The centrally mediated effects of amphetamine, methamphetamine, and MDMA.
4. The peripherally mediated effects of amphetamine, methamphetamine, and MDMA.
5. How the exchange diffusion model describes the transport of amphetamine.
6. Clinical uses of amphetamine.
7. Distinguish between amphetamine psychosis and schizophrenia.
8. Describe how neurotoxicity develops with the use of amphetamine.

Amphetamine was first synthesized in Germany in 1887, but it was not until 1927 that Gordon Alles re-synthesized and tested the compound. In 1933, Alles first described the bronchodilator and respiratory stimulant action of amphetamine. He compared the effects of amphetamine to epinephrine, noting that the cardiovascular effects of amphetamine had a longer duration of action than epinephrine.

Drugs of Abuse: Pharmacology and Molecular Mechanisms, First Edition. Sherrel G. Howard.
© 2014 John Wiley & Sons, Inc. Published 2014 by John Wiley & Sons, Inc.

INDIRECTLY ACTING SYMPATHOMIMETIC

Amphetamine and the analogs of amphetamine are in a class of drugs called "central nervous system (CNS) stimulants," and they are also referred to as indirectly acting sympathomimetics. There are two mechanisms whereby drugs can stimulate the sympathetic nervous system— direct-acting drugs or indirect-acting drugs. Amphetamine, and the analogs of amphetamine, cannot directly stimulate the neurotransmitter receptors. Therefore, they act "indirectly" by causing release of the neurotransmitter or by blocking reuptake (e.g., cocaine) thereby increasing the concentration of neurotransmitter in the synaptic cleft. Amphetamine and its analogs act indirectly to stimulate the actions of the three monoamines—dopamine (DA), norepinephrine (NE), and serotonin (5-HT). Amphetamine interacts with all of the catecholamine neuronal processes like release, reuptake, and enzymatic inactivation. The primary focus will be on the effects of amphetamine on the DA system, as the DA system produces the stimulation that leads to addiction. However, amphetamine does affect all of the catecholamines in much the same manner.

MECHANISM OF ACTION OF AMPHETAMINE

The molecular structures of DA and amphetamine are very similar (Figure 3.1). In fact, they are so similar that amphetamine is transported into the nerve terminal by a process known as Uptake I, or transport, using the DA transporter (DAT). Once inside the nerve terminal, amphetamine is taken up into the vesicles, by the vesicular uptake transporter (VMAT2), in exchange for DA, which then escapes into the cytosol (Sulzer et al., 1995). Amphetamine also acts as an inhibitor of the enzyme monoamine oxidase (MAO). Cytoplasmic MAO normally will metabolize any DA that is free in the cytoplasm; however, after inhibition by amphetamine, the intraneuronal concentration of DA increases, from DA released from the vesicles and/or from a slight decrease in the activity of MAO. This increase in the concentration of cytoplasmic DA leads to a "release" of DA using the transporter, where it can act on the postsynaptic receptor (Figure 3.2).

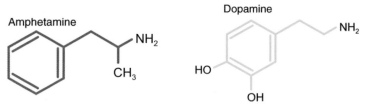

Figure 3.1   Structure of dopamine compared to d-amphetamine.

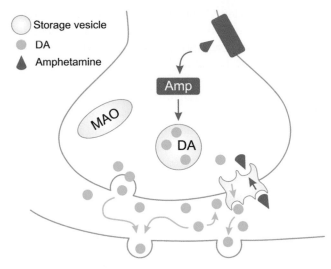

Figure 3.2   Amphetamine is taken up into the nerve ending by the transporter system.

Exocytosis is not involved in this process. There was no depolarization, and no release from vesicles. Because there was no depolarization, there is no requirement for Ca^{++}, as would be required had there been an action potential.

There are several models which have been put forth to describe the process whereby amphetamine uses the transporter to enter the nerve ending. One model is called the "exchange diffusion model" (Fisher and Cho, 1979). In this model amphetamine occupies sites on the transporter protein and is transported into the nerve ending. Since the available sites are occupied by amphetamine, DA is not inactivated by reuptake into the nerve ending and remains in the synaptic cleft. Therefore, there are only available sites on the transporter for DA to be taken out of the neuron. Basically, the carrier system is operating *in reverse* with respect to DA, namely increasing removal from the neuron and inhibiting reuptake of DA.

The second model, which is not incompatible with the exchange diffusion model, is a model where the primary site of action of amphetamine is the VMAT2 (Sulzer et al., 1995). Here, amphetamine produces a rapid increase in cytosolic DA by acting as a substrate for VMAT2. There is a decrease in vesicular DA, and a rapid increase in the concentration of DA in the presynaptic terminal. The increase in DA in the presynaptic neuron is now available to interact with the DAT, thus promoting reverse transport.

Amphetamine and the analogs of amphetamine have also been shown to demonstrate a similar effect on the serotonergic system. Namely, amphetamine interacts with the 5-HT transporter (SERT) blocking the reuptake of 5-HT, and moving 5-HT from the presynaptic neuron into the synaptic cleft via SERT. The action of amphetamine on the SERT is similar to that seen in the DA system. (Jones and Kauer, 1999; Schmitz et al., 2001).

The effect of amphetamine on the DA system is very complex and for certain mechanisms, dose dependent. The actions on presynaptic DA are well established, that is, amphetamine inhibits reuptake, inhibits MAO and therefore intraneuronal degradation of DA, activates synthesis, and depletes vesicular stores. The concentration of DA in the vesicles is known to be reduced by amphetamine, and in a recent study, Chu et al. (2010) demonstrated that amphetamine increases release of DA from the vesicles. However, the concentration of DA does not change within the nerve terminal, as might be expected, possibly due to an increase in DA synthesis as suggested by Chu et al. (2010). When reuptake is inhibited by amphetamine, it enhances the action of the newly released DA because the carrier is no longer removing the neurotransmitter from the synaptic cleft via the transport system. As long as the neurotransmitter remains in this region, it will be available to interact with the pre- and postsynaptic receptors. Since reuptake into the nerve ending is the primary means of inactivating these neurotransmitters, blocking reuptake prolongs the interaction of the neurotransmitter with the receptor. If amphetamine is occupying all sites on the transporter, DA will remain in the synaptic cleft. Therefore, amphetamine enhances the action of the "released" catecholamine by prolonging its time in the synaptic cleft.

The mechanisms of action of amphetamine are the following.

1. Amphetamine inhibits reuptake (DAT).
2. Amphetamine occupies the vesicular transporter.
3. Amphetamine partially inhibits MAO.
4. Amphetamine indirectly releases DA.

Amphetamine inhibits the reuptake of all three monoamines with varying affinities. Amphetamine and methamphetamine inhibit both the DA and the NE transporter with roughly the same affinity, while having a weaker effect on the SERT. Methylenedioxymethamphetamine (MDMA) is a unique analog of amphetamine in that it has a greater affinity for the SERT than it has for the DA or the NE transporter. Two analogs of amphetamine (methamphetamine and MDMA) will be discussed later in this chapter.

AMPHETAMINE, A PSYCHOMOTOR STIMULANT

Amphetamine is an indirectly acting sympathomimetic. This means that it mimics the effect of stimulating the sympathetic nervous system, and that it does this indirectly, as opposed to directly stimulating the DA receptor.

Drugs that produce a predominantly stimulant effect in the CNS fall into one of three categories:

1. Convulsant or respiratory stimulant
2. Psychomotor stimulant
3. Psychotomimetic drug.

Amphetamine and its analogs, as well as cocaine fall into the second category, psychomotor stimulant. While there are many amphetamine analogs, methamphetamine, methylenedioxyamphetamine (MDA), and MDMA, just to name a few, we will consider amphetamine as the prototype drug in this group. All of these drugs have some pharmacological properties in common.

While amphetamine was first synthesized as a bronchodilator, it is presently used clinically for several different disorders such as the following.

1. Obesity or to produce weight loss.
2. To treat attention deficit disorder.
3. To treat narcolepsy.

Amphetamine produces a diverse range of effects in both humans and animals. Animal and human research have demonstrated that both DA and NE play a role in behavioral disorders, obesity, schizophrenia, and drug abuse. If we first examine the central effects of amphetamine in both humans and animals, we will find that they are very similar. We will be differentiating between CENTRAL (occurring in the brain) and PERIPHERAL (occurring in the rest of the body) effects of the drugs we are studying. The central effects of amphetamine are primarily derived from amphetamine blocking the DAT and SERT, while blocking the NE transporter tends to produce more of the peripheral effects of amphetamine. DA does not play a large role in the peripheral nervous system.

CENTRAL EFFECT PRODUCED BY AMPHETAMINE

- Increased locomotor activity
- Euphoria and/or excitement
- Stereotyped behavior
- Anorexia
- Increased alertness

When large doses of amphetamine are used, a schizophrenia-like syndrome can also be produced. Amphetamines also produce peripheral sympathomimetic effects.

PERIPHERAL EFFECTS PRODUCED BY AMPHETAMINE

- Increase in blood pressure/vasoconstriction
- Increase in heart rate
- Decrease in gastrointestinal motility
- Bronchodilation

Amphetamines were very popular drugs among students in the 1960s because one could stay up all night and study and hopefully do well on your exams the next day. It was thought that amphetamine improved one's performance and memory. However, there are many stories about students who spent the entire final exam simply writing their name. It is difficult to tell if this is a "college legend" or if it is based on fact.

Many animal studies have demonstrated that amphetamine produces the following.

Increased alertness
Increased locomotor activity
Increased grooming
Increased aggressive behavior

However, exploration of novel objects by rats is reduced after amphetamine treatment. The animals move around more, but appear less aware of the environment. A normal rat will systematically explore a new environment. If the rat is put in a box, it will run around the edge of the box examining the new territory. The amphetamine-treated rat will run around more, going back and forth across the middle of the box, and although the rat is very active, it is seemingly unaware of its surroundings.

Human studies have demonstrated that amphetamine has a profound effect on motor activity, eating behavior, sleep, attention, aggression, sexual behavior, learning, and memory (Cruickshank and Dyer, 2009); all of these behaviors are similar to those seen in animal studies.

Amphetamine increases the overall rate of responding in conditioned response studies, but has not been shown to affect the conditioning process. In a fixed interval paradigm, where the animal is rewarded for pressing a lever every 10 minutes with a food pellet, there is a difference in the animal's responding pattern. A trained animal will press the lever infrequently after a food reward and increase lever pressing only toward the end of the 10-minute period, when another reward is due. Under the same conditions, the amphetamine-treated animal will continue pressing the lever after the food reward, even increasing the number of responses at the beginning of the 10-minute interval, and continue pressing the lever throughout the 10-minute interval. Under these conditions amphetamine does not improve the animal's ability to learn faster. Amphetamine does seem to simply increase the activity of the animal and the number of responses that are being measured (Butcher and Butcher, unpublished data).

With large doses of amphetamine, the animal develops stereotyped behavior. Stereotyped behavior is a behavior characterized by repeating the same behavior, over and over. In rats, this can be seen in such behaviors as licking, chewing, movement of the head and/or limbs. Amphetamine-induced stereotyped behavior takes over the behavior of the animal. Stereotyped behaviors can also be seen in Parkinson's disease patients shortly after they receive a dose of L-DOPA. Parkinson's disease is a neurological disorder characterized by a degeneration of DA neurons and a marked decrease in the concentration of DA within DA neurons. Stores of DA are somewhat replenished with a treatment of L-DOPA. One Parkinson's disease patient would pound nails in a wall (a form of stereotype behavior) after receiving his dose of L-DOPA, which would continue until the effect of the excess DA wore off. In both cases the phenomena are the result of an excess of DA or NE in the synaptic cleft.

Chronic abusers of amphetamine develop complex stereotyped behaviors consisting of meaningless behaviors that are repeated over and over, in an almost ritualized manner. This can include picking lint from clothes or other objects or a pattern of turning lights off and on. Stereotyped behaviors develop after multiple doses of amphetamine, and the behaviors seen in humans, resemble the behavior seen in animal studies.

BLOCKING THE EFFECT OF AMPHETAMINE

The action of any drug can be blocked if the mechanism of action, or even the site of action is known. Referring back to Chapter 2, consider the synthetic pathway for DA and NE, if the synthesis of the neurotransmitters are blocked or inhibited, there will be a decrease in the amount of neurotransmitter that will be available for release into the synaptic cleft. A second site to consider would be the carrier/transporter. Since amphetamine is being transported into the nerve ending, blocking the transporter will inhibit the use of the transporter by amphetamine. Additionally, when the DAT is occupied by amphetamine, the postsynaptic receptor for DA will be stimulated due to a decrease in the reuptake of DA. If the postsynaptic receptor is blocked, this will attenuate the effect of amphetamine by eliminating the site of action of the released DA. By considering drugs that will inhibit or enhance the different processes in the neuron, it is possible to increase or decrease the effects of a particular drug. Several experimental examples are listed below that demonstrate how a drug effect can be manipulated. This approach will also help you evaluate animal and clinical studies.

Animal Studies: Mechanism of Action of Amphetamine

Animal studies have shown that the behavioral effects of amphetamine are abolished by pretreatment with 6-OHDA. 6-OHDA is a neurotoxic agent that destroys the nerve endings, primarily of DA, but also NE neurons. These studies helped demonstrate that the behavioral effects produced by amphetamine are due to its effect on the neurotransmitters, DA and NE. Another method of abolishing the effect of amphetamine would be to pretreat the animal with α-methyl-para-tyrosine. α-methyl-para-tyrosine is an inhibitor of the biosynthesis of NE and DA in that it inhibits tyrosine hydroxylase (see Chapter 2). If one blocks the synthesis of a neurotransmitter, then there will be less neurotransmitter to be released into the synaptic cleft, thus decreasing the response to amphetamine. MAO inhibitors (MAO metabolizes NE and DA within the nerve ending) (see Chapter 2) would then increase the effect of amphetamine by blocking the metabolism of NE and DA within the nerve terminal.

Studies have demonstrated that some behavioral effects of amphetamine are predominantly the result of DA release. This was demonstrated in several studies. In one study, the central noradrenergic bundle was destroyed. After recovery, the animals still responded to amphetamine with an increase in locomotor activity. The responses that were affected were predominantly the result of NE release— cognition, sleep, etc. However, when the nucleus accumbens was lesioned or DA receptors were blocked pharmacologically with a neuroleptic, then the response to amphetamine was reduced or blocked (Anden et al., 1970). These animal studies helped to determine the mechanism of action of amphetamine, and would not be possible in a clinical setting.

CLINICAL USE OF AMPHETAMINE

Amphetamine has been used clinically to treat narcolepsy, obesity, attention deficit hyperactivity disorder (ADHD), some forms of Parkinson's disease, and depression.

Amphetamine as an Appetite Suppressant

Amphetamine and its analogs can produce anorexia. One of the first uses of amphetamine was as an aid to weight loss, as it reduces one's appetite and decreases food intake. However, with repeated use over time, a tolerance to amphetamine can develop and larger doses of amphetamine are required to produce the same effect. When the patient stops taking amphetamine, weight gain can and does occur in some cases. If food intake returns to the previous level of food consumption, the lost weight will return. (Obesity is a complex problem. When amphetamines are used to treat obesity, other factors should also be taken into consideration, such as mental, psychological, and physical disorders. While a tolerance to amphetamine may develop, poor eating habits and lack of exercise also contribute to the problem of obesity. Simply taking a drug will not solve this problem.)

Tolerance is the need for larger and larger doses to obtain the same effect that was initially obtained by the drug.

In some individuals amphetamine produces euphoria as the dose of amphetamine is increased. This increases the risk of amphetamine dependence.

Amphetamine as a Treatment for Narcolepsy

Narcolepsy is a neurological disorder that is characterized by excessive sleepiness and sleep attacks during the day or at inappropriate times. Amphetamine, or an analog of amphetamine, is still used in the treatment of narcolepsy. The effects of amphetamine have been demonstrated to provide a beneficial stimulant effect to patients suffering from narcolepsy (Lyon and Robbins, 1975).

Amphetamine Use as a Treatment for Attention Deficit Hyperactivity Disorder

Another beneficial use for amphetamine is in the treatment of ADHD. Children suffering from ADHD tend to have difficulty focusing for longer periods of time and often display agitated or aggressive behavior. Amphetamine in the ADHD patient increases the ability to focus and pay attention and decreases agitated behavior. In a normal well-rested child, amphetamine acts as a stimulant and may increase agitated behavior. This effect is often called a paradoxical response, because amphetamine is a stimulant in normal children, and calming in the ADHD child.

Physical and mental fatigue is reduced by amphetamine and many studies have shown that amphetamine improves performance in fatigued subjects. While low doses of amphetamine may improve performance for complicated tasks in a well-rested subject, higher doses of amphetamine do not tend to improve performance in complicated tasks. Mental performance and alertness are improved for simple tedious tasks more than for difficult tasks, which explain why truck drivers and the military often use it, when alertness for many hours is of primary importance. Similarly, amphetamine-like drugs produce a small but significant improvement in athletic performance particularly in endurance events. They are of course banned from competitions and easily detected in urine samples.

ABUSE OF AMPHETAMINE

Amphetamine or any of the amphetamine analogs are among the top five commonly abused drugs. It has been taken in pill form orally, intravenously (IV), snorted, and smoked, and depending on the route of administration, the behavioral effects of amphetamine or an analog of amphetamine can be very different. Since amphetamine and amphetamine-like stimulants have a high abuse potential, why are they so widely used? The easy answer is that the stimulants increase alertness, produce a feeling of well-being and may increase productivity.

However, in humans, amphetamine also produces euphoria. When taken by IV injection or smoked, the response can be so intense as to be described as orgasmic. Subjects in experimental studies demonstrate a more confident behavior, become hyperactive and talkative, and claim that their sex drive has increased. This does not mean that performance is enhanced, but just the desire.

Euphoria can occur even when the dose of amphetamine is low in the first-time user. In the more vulnerable individuals, the desire to intensify the drug-induced euphoria produces a need for larger and larger doses of amphetamine. This search for a more intense euphoria results in the use of higher and higher doses of the stimulant. The desire for high-dose euphoria progresses to "binge" drug use, which will eventually result in stereotyped behavior or more serious toxic effects, such as cardiovascular collapse. There is a shift from occasional use, to compulsive drug use, to high-dose binges that can last for days. Large amounts of amphetamine may be consumed during these binges with a high risk of acute toxicity, stroke, or pulmonary hypertension occurring. The demand for the drug now displaces all other considerations. The high-dose binges are followed by exhaustion, hypersomnia, social withdrawal, and depression. This withdrawal syndrome is part of the pattern of amphetamine abuse. The period of depression can last for several weeks. The withdrawal syndrome can be a period of dysphoria, or a severe depression with social withdrawal and thoughts of suicide.

AMPHETAMINE PSYCHOSIS

There are two forms of "amphetamine psychosis." There is a toxic psychosis that usually occurs after large doses, and can occur, even in first-time users. The user becomes confused and disoriented; however, they will recover from this psychosis. The second psychosis is due to repeated use and resembles schizophrenia. If amphetamine is taken repeatedly over the course of days, a state of "amphetamine psychosis" can develop. The repeated dosing occurs quite frequently as users seek to maintain the euphoric high that previously a single dose produced. The amphetamine psychosis that develops resembles an acute schizophrenic episode with hallucinations, often accompanied by paranoid symptoms and aggressive behavior. At the same time, repetitive stereotyped behavior may also develop, such as polishing shoes or head bobbing. The close similarity of this condition to schizophrenia, combined with the effectiveness of antipsychotic drugs in controlling it, contributed to the development of the DA theory of schizophrenia. Both forms of amphetamine psychosis will improve when amphetamine is cleared from the system.

Deaths do occur, which are directly related to amphetamine use. The most frequent causes are the following.

1. Cerebrovascular hemorrhage
2. Cardiovascular collapse
3. Hyperthermia
4. Bacterial endocarditis

Surprisingly, deaths occur more commonly in the occasional user, as opposed to the drug-tolerant chronic addict.

In summary, while amphetamine can prove useful in the treatment of several disorders, the euphoria and stimulation that is produced often leads to habitual use and abuse. With increasing doses and repeated use, a tolerance does develop to the enhanced mood produced by amphetamine.

TOLERANCE AND DEPENDENCE

Tolerance to and dependence on amphetamine and amphetamine analogs does develop. Tolerance develops rapidly to the euphoria and the anorexic effects of amphetamine. However, tolerance develops more slowly to some of the other effects of amphetamine, that is increased activity and stereotyped behavior. Dependence on amphetamine appears to be a consequence of avoiding the unpleasant after-effects that occur when one is coming "down" from the drug and feeling tired and lethargic. It has also been reported that the memory of the euphoria also contributes to the repeated use of amphetamine. Even a single dose of amphetamine which produces euphoria, but not acute psychotic symptoms, usually leaves the subject feeling tired and depressed when the effects of the drug have worn off. These after-effects are due to a decrease in the concentration of DA in the synaptic cleft.

One very important difference between the amphetamines and other abused drugs is that the amphetamines are neurotoxic. While the neurotoxicity may act through a glutamate receptor (Figure 3.3), possibly the NMDA receptor, the main transmitters affected are DA and 5-HT (see Chapter 2).

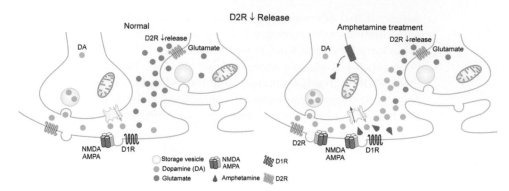

Figure 3.3   Effect of amphetamine on the interaction of dopamine and glutamate.

PHARMACOKINETICS

Amphetamine is readily absorbed, when taken orally, from the GI tract and freely penetrates the blood–brain barrier. It is also readily absorbed from the nasal mucosa and is often taken by "snorting." Some amphetamine is excreted unchanged in urine; however, since amphetamine is a weak base, the rate of excretion can be increased by making the urine more acidic. The plasma half-life of amphetamine in humans is usually about 5 hours, but it can be as long as 20–30 hours, depending on urine flow and pH. Amphetamine is metabolized by oxidative deamination. This is the primary route of biotransformation in both rabbit and man. In the rat, amphetamine is preferentially metabolized to p-hydroxyamphetamine.

METHAMPHETAMINE

Methamphetamine is a member of the phenethylamine family and exists in either a dextrorotatory or a levorotatory form (Figure 3.4). The dextrorotatory form or the racemic mixture (equal amounts of d and l) is highly addictive and a potent CNS stimulant. Its worldwide abuse can be attributed to its stimulant and euphoria-producing effects and its relatively

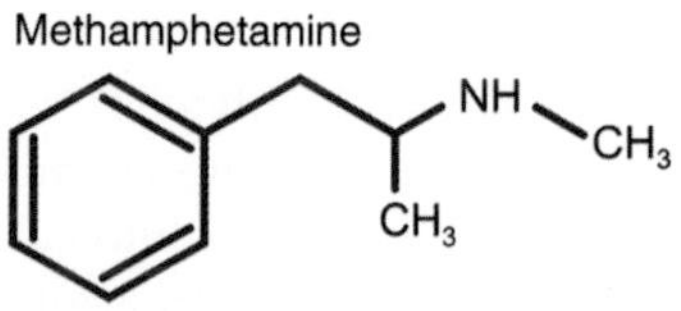

Figure 3.4   Structure of methamphetamine.

low cost. Like amphetamine it has been prescribed for weight loss, narcolepsy, and ADHD, although it is now rarely used clinically. Methamphetamine use and abuse has gone through several phases of popularity, beginning with its use during World War II, when it was given to soldiers and pilots, along with other analogs of amphetamine to increase alertness during critical maneuvers. The pharmacological properties of methamphetamine are similar to amphetamine and with the other drugs in the group of psychomotor stimulants. However, there is a difference between methamphetamine and amphetamine in that, when a comparable dose is taken, higher amounts of methamphetamine gets into the brain. Because of the additional methyl group, methamphetamine is more lipid soluble, crossing the blood–brain barrier more quickly. It is therefore a more potent stimulant when compared to amphetamine.

Methamphetamine is known by many other names, the most common is ice, but crank, speed, and crystal are also common. The trade names for methamphetamine are many—Methedrine, Desoxyn, Dexoval, Dexyfed, Efroxine, Norodin, Stemoxydine, Syndrox, and this is not a complete list.

CENTRAL AND PERIPHERAL EFFECTS

Methamphetamine is a psychomotor stimulant, and like amphetamine, the main central effects are the following.

1. Locomotor stimulation
2. Euphoria or excitement
3. Stereotyped behavior
4. Anorexia

The primary peripheral nervous system effects produced by methamphetamine include the following.

1. Increase in blood pressure
2. Increase in heart rate
3. Decrease in gastrointestinal motility
4. Bronchodilation

These effects are the same as those found after amphetamine ingestion.

CLINICAL USES FOR METHAMPHETAMINE

Methamphetamine was first used as a bronchodilator to manage asthma symptoms. In the 1930s it was also used to manage schizophrenia, morphine addiction, and hypotension. Amphetamine inhalers were available without prescription until 1960. After 1960, methamphetamine was only available by prescription for depression, heroin addiction, and obesity.

Because of the known stimulating action in the CNS, it was hoped that methamphetamine could be used to alleviate the slowness or lack of motor activity in Parkinson patients. Secondarily, it was thought it would be useful in combating the sedation that resulted from the large doses of anticholinergics that were commonly used in the treatment of Parkinson's disease. Unfortunately, very little improvement was noted. Although methamphetamine slightly reduced the rigidity of Parkinson's disease, and there was a slight improvement in motor performance, it was not consistently effective in all patients. Basically, methamphetamine was only good for use in one type of Parkinson's disease patient namely, postencephalitic parkinsonism, and occasionally it also worked for slower, overly sedated patients.

Amphetamine and methamphetamine were examined with respect to their potential value in treating depression. It would seem that a drug that produces euphoria might be useful in treating depression. However, amphetamines were only effective in a small population of depressed patients, and only in patients with mild or moderate depression. Neither drug was found useful in treating severe depression.

Epinephrine and ephedrine were the first adrenergic drugs. Many of their derivatives and substitutes have since come into general use. Ideally any substitute should have an advantage therapeutically over any drug it replaces. Or else why replace it? A rule of thumb when examining the structure of a compound would be:

The structure of a compound determines the type of adrenergic action possessed by the amine and similarly determines the therapeutic use, as well as the side effects.

If one assumes that epinephrine or ephedrine have the optimal chemical structure when comparing adrenergic drugs, then, the structure–activity relationship of a new drug would be compared to epinephrine or ephedrine. In comparing amphetamine and methamphetamine with ephedrine, methamphetamine is more potent than amphetamine with respect to its central stimulant properties because it is more lipophilic and will get into the brain more quickly. While both amphetamine and methamphetamine use the monoamine transporter systems of all three biogenic amines, DA (DAT), NE (NAT), and 5-HT (SERT) to exert an effect in both the central and peripheral nervous system, methamphetamine can also enter a neuron by diffusion. Methamphetamine has been shown to release more DA than amphetamine. This may be a result of its increased lipophilicity, since it uses both the DAT and diffusion to enter the DA neuron (Goodwin et al., 2009). While it is no longer used as a pressor agent, methamphetamine is more potent than ephedrine.

Methamphetamine has potentially three therapeutic uses.

1. As a CNS stimulant (treating narcolepsy, ADHD, and obesity)
2. As a pressor agent
3. A weak solution could be used as a nasal decongestant.

However, the abuse potential for methamphetamine is so high, it is rarely used clinically.

METHAMPHETAMINE ABUSE

Methamphetamine is cheap and readily available. It increases both energy and libido, decreases appetite, and enhances the mood. Methamphetamine can be snorted, taken orally, smoked, or injected. Methamphetamine is used as a recreational drug because of its stimulant and euphoria-producing effects. The route of administration will alter the onset of drug action and the effect of the drug. If the drug is smoked or injected there is an immediate "rush," followed by a feeling of extreme euphoria. Methamphetamine is commonly taken in a binge and crash cycle, meaning the drug is taken again, as soon as the euphoria starts to decline. This occurs before methamphetamine has been metabolized and left the body, so that the concentration of methamphetamine in the system continues to increase. As tolerance to the drug develops, increases in the dosage become necessary. In order to maintain the euphoria, the user will "tweak" the drug, trying to maintain the same "high." This form of binging is called a "run," and can go on for several days without food or sleep. This part of the chronic abuse cycle is physiologically the most dangerous as the greatest damage can be done to major organ systems and the brain. In 2009 in Los Angeles, over 20% of admissions to emergency rooms was the result of methamphetamine overdose. The commonly seen symptoms of methamphetamine use, some more life threatening than others, are shown in Table 3.1.

Methamphetamine effects have also been compared with those of cocaine. Although they are not structurally similar, they do have some effects in common. The effects of methamphetamine and cocaine are compared in the chart below (Table 3.2).

CLINICAL STUDY IN JAPAN

Methamphetamine, over the counter, use in Japan first occurred after World War II and peaked in 1957. At this time methamphetamine was legal and was produced by a pharmaceutical company in Japan. At the height of the first epidemic, more than 55 000 people were arrested by

Table 3.1   The Negative Clinical Symptoms That Are
Commonly Seen in Short-Term Methamphetamine Users

Dilated pupils
Dry mouth—leading to profound tooth decay,
    "MethMouth"
Elevated blood pressure and increase in heart rate
Decrease in oxygen to the extremities from poor
    circulation (leading to itchy, bleeding skin lesions)
Increase in temperature of internal organs
Decrease in appetite
Paranoia
Hyperactivity
Hyperthermia
Irritability
Anorexia
Increase in libido
Nausea/vomiting
Hallucinations (visual and auditory)
Cardiac arrhythmias
Aggression
Itching (illusion that bugs are crawling on the skin)
Stroke

the police, and there were more than half-a-million people using methamphetamine at the time.

Japan has had three separate epidemics of methamphetamine use.
These case histories are important because methamphetamine was the
only drug used by the subjects in this study, as opposed to the "cocktails"
that are more commonly used in the United States. The data compiled by

Table 3.2   Comparison of Methamphetamine and Cocaine

Methamphetamine	vs.	Cocaine
Stimulant		Stimulant and local anesthetic
Man-made		Plant-derived
Smoking produces a long-lasting high		Smoking produces a brief high
50% of drug removed from the body in 12 hours		50% removed from body in 1 hour
Increases DA release and blocks		Blocks DA reuptake
Limited medical use		Limited medical use in some surgical procedures as a local anesthetic
Dose-dependent neurotoxicity		Not known to be neurotoxic

Source: Adapted from NIDA Notes.

Ujike and Sato (2004) elucidates the long-term effect of methamphetamine, without the contamination of any other drugs or alcohol, which is difficult to obtain in studies on drug abuse.

Ujike and Sato (2004) present the case histories of three chronic methamphetamine users over a period of time. In all three cases, the subjects displayed paranoia, visual and/or auditory hallucinations, that ended with violent attacks on family members, police, and even themselves. The study provides a unique look into the use and effects of methamphetamine, without the contamination from other drugs or alcohol that is so common in drug studies.

SHORT-TERM EFFECTS OF METHAMPHETAMINE

Clinical evaluation of the effects of methamphetamine demonstrates that it stimulates the CNS. It is a powerful stimulant and can increase alertness and physical activity and decrease appetite. The most common short-term effects of methamphetamine are the following.

1. Increase in attention
2. Decrease in fatigue
3. Euphoria
4. Increase in respiration
5. Hyperthermia

TOLERANCE AND DEPENDENCE

Tolerance does develop to methamphetamine and increasingly greater doses are required to achieve the same "high." On withdrawal of methamphetamine, the addict becomes depressed, anxious, fatigued, develops paranoia and aggressive behavior, and has a severe craving for the drug. The severity of the withdrawal symptoms is dependent on the duration and amount of methamphetamine used. While there is a decrease in extracellular DA and DA metabolites (that has been demonstrated in animal studies) intraneuronal concentrations appear to be in normal range (Robinson et al., 1990). The increased release of DA does produce an increase in extracellular DA that inhibits DA neuron firing via the activation of autoreceptors and thereby blunts phasic DA neurotransmission (Branch and Beckstead, 2012). There is a decrease in the number of DA neurons in the brain. Similarly, there is also a reduction of 5-HT neurons. The neurotoxic effects of methamphetamine, as well as amphetamine and MDMA have been clearly demonstrated in animal studies (Romanelli and Smith, 2006). Whether there are neurotoxic effects in humans still remain controversial.

METABOLISM

The molecular structure of amphetamine and methamphetamine are very similar. They are both weak bases, so that acidifying the urine will increase their removal from the system. The half-life of methamphetamine can vary, as does the half-life of amphetamine, depending on the route of administration, hydration, and kidney function. Metabolism is primarily by N-demethylation to amphetamine, which is followed by oxidative deamination. The conversion to amphetamine and then deamination explains why it has a longer half-life than amphetamine.

METHYLENEDIOXYMETHAMPHETAMINE

3,4-Methylenedioxymethamphetamine (MDMA) was synthesized in Germany in 1912 by Merck Pharmaceuticals; however, it was virtually forgotten until the 1950s when the army became interested in its use as a truth serum (Figure 3.5). During the 1960s A. Schulgrin, experimenting on himself and determined that MDMA was a psychedelic drug. By the 1970s, MDMA was discovered by psychotherapists and used clinically. At this time it was considered to be a new and "safe" drug. Clinically, it was thought to help patients "open-up" or feel empathy. This was thought to improve the psychoanalytic process, so that in 1984 when the DEA proposed scheduling MDMA many psychiatrists testified against the scheduling, claiming that MDMA was not a true hallucinogen. In 1985, MDMA was classified as a Schedule I drug (MDMA: Compound raises medical, legal issues, Brain/Mind Bulletin April 15, 1985).

In the early 1980s, MDMA (ecstasy) was discovered by the "Rave" and "Club" groups. At this time the rate of adolescent drug use was relatively stable over the last few decades. By 2007, ecstasy became the third most commonly abused drug (Johnston et al., 2007) and the rate among adolescents and young adults was higher than in the general population (Substance Abuse and Mental Health Services Administration, 2009). MDMA users reported that they were "experimenting" with the drug, or that it was taken to feel good or as an aid in social interactions (Wu et al., 2010).

Methlylene dioxymethamphetamine (MDMA)

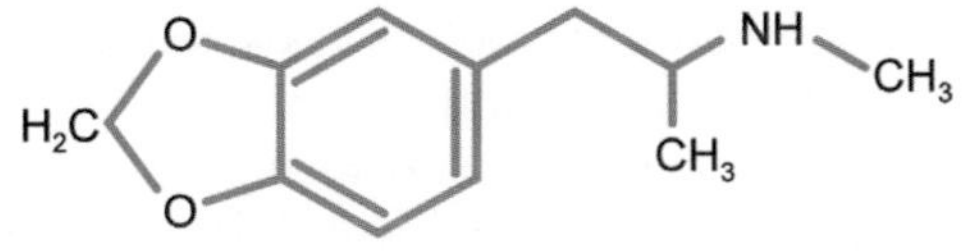

Figure 3.5   Structural formula for methylenedioxymethamphetamine (MDMA).

MDMA is presently the fourth most popular recreational drug. While it is reported by users to produce a sense of closeness or "empathy," it also has a number of other side effects, some more dangerous than others.

MECHANISM OF ACTION OF METHYLENEDIOXYMETHAMPHETAMINE

Amphetamine, methamphetamine, and MDMA have many properties in common. They enhance release of neurotransmitters, and they are all substrates for the associated transporters of DA, NE, and 5-HT. Methamphetamine and MDMA may diffuse into the nerve terminal, or be taken up by the transporter system. Additionally, the amphetamines also release glutamate (GLU) and this may account for the neurotoxicity of the amphetamines (Nash and Yamamoto, 1992). While all of the amphetamines affect the three biogenic amine transporter systems, they vary in their affinity for the different systems. MDMA has a greater affinity for the SERT than for the DAT. MDMA, much like amphetamine, produces an increase in the release of DA into the synaptic cleft and MDMA also induces an acute and rapid release of 5-HT. This combination of effects on multiple neurotransmitters produces a response that is more similar to those obtained from some of the hallucinogens (see Chapter 2 for 5-HT-Glu interaction).

CENTRAL EFFECTS OF METHYLENEDIOXYMETHAMPHETAMINE

MDMA produces a rapid increase in release of DA and 5-HT in the CNS. This rapid release of DA and 5-HT produces

1. an increase in locomotor activity;
2. a dose-dependent increase in body temperature (hyperthermia);
3. increased alertness and motivation.

While most of these CNS effects are the same for all of the amphetamine analogs, the increase in body temperature produced by MDMA is potentially fatal. MDMA also produces a syndrome called the serotonin syndrome that will be discussed later. While MDMA is thought to be a new and relatively safe drug, it is far from being a benign drug. Listed below, in Table 3.3 are some of the withdrawal effects that last for at least a week after the last dose of MDMA.

These effects mentioned in Table 3.3 can have a negative impact on one's life, but they are not life threatening. However, even with limited use of MDMA, taking into account the circumstance under which MDMA is

Table 3.3   Acute Withdrawal Effects of MDMA

Anxiety	Lack of appetite
Irritability	Decrease in libido
Impulsivity	Decrease in mental ability
Aggression	Decrease in cognitive ability
Depression	Insomnia

used (i.e., clubs or rave parties) hyperthermia can and does occur. Hyper-thermia is extremely dangerous and medical attention should be obtained promptly as hyperthermia can lead to muscle breakdown, which can, in turn lead to kidney failure. Additional symptoms that occur with MDMA are chills, nausea, sweating, dehydration, high blood pressure, and heart and kidney failure.

There is a large body of evidence that demonstrates a range of neuropsy-chiatric problems depending on the degree of recreational use of MDMA (Parrott, 2006). The occasional user of MDMA may remain unimpaired, or only suffer mild impairment, while the heavy user could suffer from cog-nitive impairment, memory loss, sleep disturbance, sexual dysfunction, a compromised immune system, and increased oxidative stress, to name a few of the problems (Parrott, 2006). While the effects of polydrug use by many users of MDMA confound these data, it should not be seen as the "safe" drug it was once thought to be. A recent study has demonstrated cognitive impairment from the long-term use of MDMA with the mini-mal use of additional drugs (Halpern et al., 2011). However, the majority of MDMA users also use a wide variety of other drugs, including stimu-lants, hallucinogens, opiates, and CNS depressants (Scholey et al., 2004); so the supporters of MDMA tend to blame the other drugs.

NEUROTOXICITY

While MDMA was once considered to be a "safe" non-addicting drug, recent studies examining the neurotoxic effects of MDMA in both ani-mal and humans have produced some conflicting data. Neurotoxic ef-fects from MDMA have been demonstrated in rodents and nonhuman pri-mates. The neurotoxic effects of MDMA in humans are still controversial; however, a recent study using positron emission tomography has demon-strated long-lasting alterations in the 5-HT 2A receptor (Parrott, 2012; 2013) that do not return to normal with abstinence. The authors concluded "given the widespread recreational popularity of this drug (MDMA), the results have critical health implications."

In both rodents and nonhuman primates, a single large dose or multi-ple large doses, will produce long-lasting deficits in the markers for both

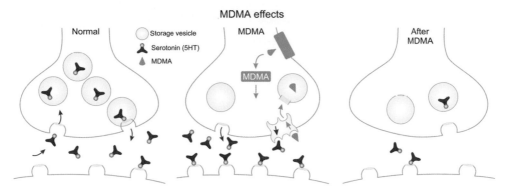

Figure 3.6   Comparison of short- and long-term effects of methylenedioxymethamphetamine (MDMA).

the DA and the 5-HT systems. This includes the levels of the neurotransmitters, the biosynthetic enzymes, receptors, and transporters (Commins et al., 1987). There is some recovery of 5-HT stores within 24 hours, but cerebral concentrations then decrease due to more specific neurotoxic damage to the 5-HT nerve endings in the forebrain. This neurodegeneration can last for months in rats and years in primates. However, the neurotoxic effect of MDMA in humans is still controversial (Kish et al., 2000). Selective long-term loss of DA nerve endings has been reported only in mice (Johnson et al., 2002). It has been suggested that this loss is due to the formation of free radicals. Evidence for the occurrence of MDMA-induced free radical formation and subsequent neurotoxic damage in humans remains equivocal. Histological data seem to demonstrate neurotoxic damage in brains of heavy MDMA users (McCann et al., 2000; Lyles and Cadet, 2003). However, most MDMA users have also used many other drugs; therefore, it is difficult to determine if the neurotoxic damage to the brain can be solely attributed to MDMA. In Figure 3.6 the acute and long-term effects of MDMA on the 5-HT neurons are shown. The acute effects of MDMA are shown in the middle figure, demonstrating the massive release of 5-HT. Long-term effects of MDMA show a marked decrease in 5-HT stores and release. When MDMA is withdrawn, a variety of negative effects are produced (Figure 3.7).

While the neurotoxic effects of MDMA seen in animals have not been consistently demonstrated in humans, Steinkellner et al. (2011) have reviewed the human data, pointing out four key mechanisms that would contribute to neurotoxicity in humans (Figure 3.3). The four effects are the following.

1. Hyperthermia
2. Metabolism of MDMA
3. Oxidative stress
4. Dysregulation of energy metabolism via mitochondria dysfunction.

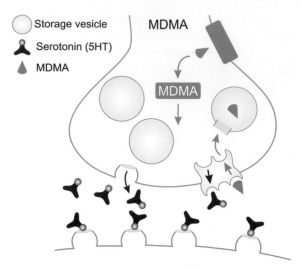

Figure 3.7   Effect of MDMA on the 5-HT neuron.

While the effects of oxidative stress, after even a single dose of MDMA, has been established for some time (Green et al., 2003; Yamamoto et al., 2010) the consequences of metabolic dysregulation are still not clear. Steinkellner et al. (2011) point out that like other amphetamines, MDMA may also be addicting and that the rewarding properties of MDMA may be accounted for by the release of DA from the mesocorticolimbic DA system.

STRUCTURES RICH IN SEROTONIN

The response to stimulating 5-HT receptors is extremely complex, primarily because there are so many 5-HT receptors. The 5-HT receptors are G protein-coupled receptors, with the exception of the 5-HT3 receptor, which is a ligand-gated ion channel receptor. In Table 3.4, there is a list

Table 3.4   5-HT Family of Receptors

Family	Type	Effect	Response
5-HT1	Gi/Go-protein coupled	Decrease cAMP	Inhibit
5-HT2	Gq/G11-protein-coupled	Increase cAMP	Excite
5-HT3	Ligand-gated Na+/K+ channel	Depolarizing	Excite
5-HT4	Gs-protein-coupled	Increase cAMP	Excite
5-HT5	Gi/Go-protein-coupled	Decrease cAMP	Inhibit
5-HT6	Gs-protein-coupled	Increase cAMP	Excite
5-HT7	Gs-protein-coupled	Increase cAMP	Excite

Source: Adapted from Hoyer et al. (1994).

of the seven different members of the 5-HT receptor family and the responses they produce. Within each family of receptors are subtypes, thus increasing further the variety of responses that can be produced by the 5-HT neurotransmitter system.

If we consider some of the effects of 5-HT stimulation or inhibition on the structures rich in 5-HT, we will be better able to predict the effects of MDMA, and to a lesser degree that of MDMA, on individual systems.

Gastrointestinal Tract

5-HT produces an increase in GI motility and contraction of isolated strips of intestines. (This is partly a direct effect on smooth muscle cells and partly an effect on enteric neurons.) Smooth muscle contracts in response to 5-HT stimulation in most animals, but produces only a minor response in smooth muscle in humans.

Blood Vessels

The effect of 5-HT on blood vessels depends on several factors—the size of the blood vessel, the species of animal, and the prevailing sympathetic tone.

Large vessels constrict: This is a direct effect on vascular smooth muscle mediated through 5-HT2A receptors.

However, 5-HT will also cause vasodilatation by acting on 5-HT1 receptors. This occurs by the following two pathways.

1. By releasing NO
2. By inhibiting NE release.

If 5-HT is injected IV, the blood pressure first rises (constriction) and then falls (dilation); this is very similar to that when NE is injected.

Platelets

5-HT causes platelet aggregation. (This is an important consideration in vascular disease).

Nerve Endings

5-HT stimulates pain-mediating sensory nerve endings by stimulating 5-HT3 receptors.

CENTRAL NERVOUS SYSTEM

As with most neurotransmitters in the CNS, 5-HT acts both pre- and post-synaptically, to excite or inhibit transmission.

ACUTE EFFECTS OF METHYLENEDIOXYMETHAMPHETAMINE

Release and Depletion of Serotonin

When one administers an acute dose of MDMA, it produces an acute and rapid release of 5-HT. The 5-HT concentration in the brain decreases markedly during the first few hours after MDMA and there is an increase in extracellular 5-HT (5-HT outside of the neuron), particularly in areas like the striatum or the prefrontal cortex. This increase in extracellular 5-HT can be attenuated by pretreating with an uptake inhibitor. A 5-HT uptake inhibitor, such as fluoxetine (Prozac) has been found to block the uptake of MDMA into the neuron by the SERT, thereby decreasing the release of 5-HT. This is the same mechanism that was discussed above for amphetamine. The data, demonstrating that a 5-HT uptake inhibitor can block the effects of MDMA, supports the hypothesis that the effects of MDMA involve a carrier-mediated mechanism. Unlike amphetamine, MDMA can diffuse into the neuron, such that blocking the transporter may not completely abolish the effects of MDMA.

Methylenedioxymethamphetamine Effects on the Serotonin System

1. MDMA is transported into the neuron by means of the 5-HT carrier.
2. MDMA inhibits tryptophan hydroxylase, the rate-limiting step in the 5-HT synthetic pathway.
3. MDMA inhibits reuptake of 5-HT.
4. MDMA increases release of 5-HT.

METHYLENEDIOXYMETHAMPHETAMINE EFFECTS ON TRYPTOPHAN HYDROXYLASE (ANIMAL STUDIES)

Tryptophan hydroxylase is inhibited by MDMA. Since tryptophan hydroxylase is the rate-limiting step in the synthesis of the amount of 5-HT synthesized will be reduced, while at the same time the neuron is releasing the available stores of 5-HT.

Tryptophan hydroxylase activity starts to decrease within 15 minutes after an acute injection of MDMA. Tryptophan hydroxylase is still reduced more than 2 weeks following a single dose of MDMA. If a tyrosine hydroxylase inhibitor depletes central DA content, then the administered MDMA-induced reduction in tryptophan hydroxylase activity will not be as great. This treatment provides a partial block.

If MDMA is applied directly into the brain, for example, in the cortex or the striatum, there is no effect on tryptophan hydroxylase activity.

One possible explanation for this finding would be that when MDMA is injected systemically, an active metabolite of MDMA is formed in the periphery, and it is this active metabolite that is responsible for the acute neurochemical effects of MDMA. One possible candidate would be MDA.

The MDMA-induced decrease in tryptophan hydroxylase activity is influenced by body temperature. If an animal is treated with MDMA at room temperature (25°C) then MDMA produces hyperthermia. However, if the room temperature is reduced to 6°C then a hypothermic response is produced. Tryptophan hydroxylase was reduced in the cortex and striatum of the hyperthermic animals, but tryptophan hydroxylase activity was not altered in the hypothermic animals.

MDMA also inhibits MAO activity. This is similar to the other amphetamine analogs that we have previously discussed. Reduction of MAO reduces the metabolism of 5-HT and DA within the nerve terminal, thereby contributing to the active release/transport of the neurotransmitters from the nerve terminal.

Release and Depletion of Dopamine after Methylenedioxymethamphetamine

MDMA also releases DA. This would be expected since it is an amphetamine analog. Analogs of a particular compound maintain many of the basic characteristics of the prototype compound.

The peak release of DA was measured using *in vivo* dialysis in the neostriatum of the rat. Peak release occurred at 120 minutes, returning to the baseline after 180 minutes. These studies were performed in the awake and freely moving animal. It has been suggested that MDMA enters DA terminals by diffusion rather than by the uptake carrier. This is supported by data which demonstrate that neither MDMA nor methamphetamine release of DA is blocked by a DA reuptake inhibitor.

MDMA does increase the formation of hydroxy radicals in the brain. This was established by measuring the oxidation of salicylate to dihydroxybenzoic acid (Liu et al., 1997; Themann et al., 2001). It has long been known that the conversion of salicylate to dihydroxybenzoic acid only occurs in the presence of hydroxy radicals; less reactive free radicals will not produce the same conversion (Themann et al., 2001). In the presence of MDMA, salicylate is converted to dihydroxybenzoic acid (Liu et al., 1997).

Aggregation Toxicity

Aggregation toxicity has been known for some time to increase the toxicity of MDMA. While it has not been demonstrated in humans, it does exist in rats and mice. Animals housed in groups, who are then treated with MDMA, demonstrated an enhanced toxicity to MDMA. This increase in toxicity was not due to over crowding, as the animals were placed in very large cages, with more space than they might have had in a single cage. Even under these conditions there was an elevated toxicity. Toxicity to MDMA was also enhanced by elevated temperature, noise, and poor hydration. One cannot help wondering if the toxicity is increased at the rave parties held in the deserts of California. Here there would be an increase in the number of people, noise, dehydration, and temperature.

METHYLENEDIOXYMETHAMPHETAMINE AND THE SEROTONIN SYNDROME

MDMA produces a rapid increase in the release of 5-HT and DA in the CNS, as mentioned above. As a result of these two transmitters being rapidly released there is not only an increase in activity and an increase in temperature, but also a behavioral response called the serotonin syndrome. Behavioral effects of the serotonin syndrome in rats or mice include:

1. Hyperactivity	5. Penile erection
2. Ejaculation	6. Head weaving-bobbing
3. Piloerection	7. Forepaw treading
4. Salivation	8. Defecation

After an acute injection of MDMA a slight recovery of the 5-HT stores can be seen in the CNS within the first 24 hours. However, the cerebral concentration of 5-HT begins to decline, due to specific neurotoxic damage to the 5-HT nerve endings in the forebrain. This neurodegeneration can last for months in rats and for years in primates. In mice, one can also see a selective long-term loss of DA nerve endings. This may be due to the formation of free radicals, which we mentioned earlier.

HALLUCINOGENIC EFFECTS OF METHYLENEDIOXYMETHAMPHETAMINE

MDMA usually produces a relaxed, euphoric state, including emotional openness, empathy, reduction of negative thoughts, and decrease in inhibition. Sounds and colors can appear more intense, which is the reason for the classification as a hallucinogen or psychedelic drug. When one considers hallucinogenic drugs, one usually thinks of lysergic acid diethylamide (LSD) as a prototype drug. Most of the drugs that are included among the psychedelics are related in some way to the indolealkylamines, that is, 5-HT.

All drugs are put into specific categories, usually defined by structure and activity. As an example, a drug like LSD is included among the drugs listed as psychedelics. Most drugs listed as "psychedelics" are related to the indolealkylamines, that is, 5-HT. Description of a response to a psychedelic drug would include several major effects. Responses as reported by users of psychedelic drugs are the following.

1. Heighted awareness of sensory input
2. A feeling that "self" is divided, spectator self and participating self
3. The environment is novel and beautiful
4. Attention may be turned inward
5. Everything/anything takes on a great meaning or sense of truth.

Commonly there is a diminished capacity in their ability to determine boundaries between people and objects. The ability to differentiate the boundaries of any two objects or people may be what produces the reported feelings of union with all of mankind.

There are three criteria for categorizing LSD-type drugs.

1. Subjective effects
2. Cross-tolerance between compounds
3. Response to selective antagonists.

MDMA falls into the category of LSD-like, but with other properties. There is no cross-tolerance between LSD and the amphetamines and because of this, MDMA is rather in a category of its own. The combination of MDMA with LSD will be discussed in Chapter 9.

REINSTATEMENT

Reinstatement of drug-seeking behavior is a problem with the psychomotor stimulants. One primary reason is that the drug user of amphetamine or methamphetamine always remembers the euphoria or the "high," the self-confidence, and one's seemingly endless energy. Drug therapy has not been as successful with the amphetamines as with other abused drugs. MDMA, previously considered to be a "safe" recreational drug, has recently been shown to act as a primer for behavior previously maintained by amphetamine (McClung et al., 2010) suggesting that MDMA-seeking behavior and amphetamine-seeking behavior have common cues. While MDMA may be a weaker reinforcer compared to methamphetamine (Lile et al., 2005; Wang and Woolverton, 2007), nonetheless, MDMA and the MDMA-associated cues do reinstate drug-seeking behavior in some animals (Ball et al., 2007). These studies share important similarities with clinical studies in that they point out that certain individuals are more vulnerable than others and with longer drug usage the difference in the vulnerable individual becomes more obvious.

PHARMACOKINETICS IN HUMANS

MDMA is well absorbed orally. The novice user will usually consume 1–2 tablets, and more experienced users can consume three or more tablets per session. This difference does imply a development of tolerance. Heavy users do go on amphetamine-like binges in an attempt to continue the initial high. These binges can last for several days.

Pharmacokinetic Properties

Onset of action	20–60 minutes
Peak effect	60–90 minutes
Duration of Action	~5 hours

Review Questions

1. Describe how neurotoxicity develops when using amphetamine.
2. Why is the dependence potential so high with amphetamine?
3. What is the difference between the central effects of amphetamine and MDMA?
4. Why is MDMA not the "safe drug" that it was once thought to be?
5. Why are the effects of MDMA so widespread?
6. Describe the serotonin syndrome.
7. Is MDMA a psychedelic drug, and if so why?

REFERENCES AND ADDITIONAL READING

Anden NE, Butcher SG, Corrodi H, Fuxe K, Ungerstedt U. 1970. Receptor activity and turnover of dopamine and noradrenaline after neuroleptics. *Eur. J. Pharmacol.* 11:303–314.

Ball KT, Walsh KM, Rebec GV. 2007. Reinstatement of MDMA (ecstasy) seeking by exposure to discrete drug-conditioned cues. *Pharm. Biochem. Behav.* 87:420–425.

Branch SY, Beckstead MJ. 2012. Methamphetamine produces bidirectional, concentration-dependent effects on dopamine neuron excitability and dopamine-mediated synaptic currents. *J. Neurophysiol.* 108:802–809.

Chu PW, Hadlock GC, Vieira-Brock P, Stout K, Hanson GR, Fleckenstein AE. 2010. Methamphetamine alters vesicular monoamine transporter-2 function and potassium-stimulated dopamine release. *J Neurochem.* 115:325–332.

Commins DL, Vosmer G, Virus RM, Woolverton WL, Schuster CR, Seiden LS. 1987. Biochemical and histological evidence that methylenedioxymethylamphetamine (MDMA) is toxic to neurons in the rat brain. *J. Pharmacol. Exp. Ther.* 241:338–345.

Cruickshank DC, Dyer KR. 2009. A review of the clinical pharmacology of methamphetamine. *Addiction.* 104:1084–1099.

Fischer JF, Cho AK. 1979. Chemical release of dopamine from striatal homogenates: evidence for an exchange diffusion model. *J. Pharmacol. Exp. Ther.* 208:203–209.

Goodwin JS, Larson GA, Swant J, et al. 2009. Amphetamine and methamphetamine differentially affect dopamine transporters in vitro and in vivo. *J. Biol. Chem.* 284:2978–2989.

Green AR, Mechan AO, Elliott JM, O'Shea E, Colado MI. 2003. The pharmacology and clinical pharmacology of 3,4-methlenedioxymethamphetamine (MDMA, 'ecstasy'). *Pharmacol. Rev.* 55:463–508.

Halpern JH, Sherwood AR, Hudson JI, Gruber S, Kozin D, Pope HG Jr. 2011. Residual neurocognitive features of long-term ecstasy users with minimal exposure to other drugs. *Addiction.* 106:777–786.

Hoyer D, Clarke DE, Fozard JR, et al. 1994. International Union of Pharmacology classification of receptors for 5-hydroxytryptamine (serotonin). *Pharmacol. Rev.* 46:157–203.

Johnson EA, O'Callaghan JP, Miller DB. 2002. Chronic treatment with supraphysiological levels of corticosterone enhances D-MDMA-induced dopaminergic neurotoxicity in the C57BL/6J female mouse. *Brain Res.* 933:130–138.

Johnston LD, O'Malley PM, Bachman JG, Schulenberg JE. 2007. Monitoring the future national survey results on drug use: 1975–2006. Volume I: *Secondary School Students 2006.* National Institute on Drug Abuse, Bethesda, MD.

Jones S, Kauer JA. 1999. Amphetamine depresses excitatory synaptic transmission via serotonin receptors in the ventral tegmental area. *J. Neurosci.* 19:9780–9787.

Kish SJ, Furukawa Y, Ang L, Vorce SP, Kalasinsky KS. 2000. Striatal serotonin is depleted in brain of a human MDMA (Ecstasy) user. *Neurology.* 55:294–296.

Lile JA, Ross JT, Nader MA. 2005. A comparison of the reinforcing efficacy of 3,4-methylenedioxymethamphetamine (MDMA, "ecstasy") with cocaine in rhesus monkeys. *Drug Alcohol Depend.* 78:135–140.

Liu L, Leech JA, Urch RB, Silverman FS. 1997. In vivo salicylate hydroxylation: a potential biomarker for assessing acute ozone exposure and effects in humans. *Am. J. Respir. Crit. Care Med.* 156:1405–1412.

Lyles J, Cadet JL. 2003. Methylenedioxymethamphetamine (MDMA, Ecstasy) neurotoxicity: cellular and molecular mechanisms. *Brain Res. Rev.* 42:155–168.

Lyon M, Robbins T. 1975. The action of central nervous system stimulant drugs: a general theory concerning amphetamine effects. In: Essman WB,

Valzelli L (eds), *Current Developments in Psychopharmacology*. Spectrum, New York.

McCann UD, Eligulashvili V, Ricaurte GA. 2000. (+/-) 3,4-Methylenedioxymethamphetamine (Ecstasy)-induced serotonin neurotoxicity: clinical studies. *Neuropsychobiology*. 42:11–16.

McClung J, Fantegrossi W, Howell L. 2010. Reinstatement of extinguished amphetamine self administration by 3,4-methylenedioxymethamphetamine (MDMA) and its enantiomers in rhesus monkeys. *Psychopharmacology (Berl)*. 210:75–83l.

Nash JF and Yamamoto BK. 1992. Methamphetamine neurotoxicity and striatal glutamate release: comparison to 3,4-methylenedioxymethamphetamine. *Brain Res*. 58:237–243.

Parrott AC. 2006. MDMA in humans: factors which affect the neuropsychobiological profiles of recreational ecstasy users, the integrative role of bioenergetic stress. *Psychopharmcol*. 20:147–163.

Parrott AC. 2012. MDMA and 5-HT neurotoxicity: the empirical evidence for its adverse effects in humans-no need for translation. *Br. J Pharmacol*. 166:1518–1520.

Parrott, AC. 2013. Human psychobiology of MDMA or "Ecstasy": an overview of 25 years of empirical research. *Hum. Psychopharmacol*. 28:2289–2307.

Robinson TE, Yew J, Paulson PE, Camp DM. 1990. The long-term effects of neurotoxic doses of methamphetamine on the extracellular concentration of dopamine measured with microdialysis in striatum. *Neurosci. Lett*. 110:193–198.

Romanelli F, Smith KM. 2006. Clinical effects and management of methamphetamine abuse. *Pharmacotherapy*. 26:1148–1156.

Schmitz Y, Lee C, Schmauss C, Gonon F, Sulzer D. 2001. Amphetamine distorts stimulation-dependent dopamine overflow: effects on D2 auto receptors, transporters and synaptic vesicle stores. *J. Neurosci*. 21:5916–5924.

Scholey AB, Parrott AC, Buchanan T, Heffernan T, Ling J, Rodgers J. 2004. Increased intensity of ecstasy and polydrug usage in the more experienced recreational ecstasy/MDMA users: a www study. *Addictive Behav*. 29:743–752.

Steinkellner T, Freissmuth M, Sitte HH, Montgomery T. 2011. The ugly side of amphetamines: short- and long-term toxicity of 3,4-methylenedioxymethamphetamine (MDMA, 'Ecstasy'), methamphetamine and D-amphetamine. *Biol. Chem*. 392:103–115.

Sulzer D, Chen T, Lau Y, Kristensen H, Rayport S, Ewing A. 1995. Amphetamine redistributes dopamine from synaptic vesicles to the cytosol and promotes reverse transport. *J. Neurosci*. 15:4102–4108.

Themann C, Teismann P, Kuschinsky K, Ferger B. 2001. Comparison of two independent aromatic hydroxylation assays in combination with intracerebral microdialysis to determine hydroxyl free radicals. *J. Neurosci. Methods*. 108:57–64.

Ujike H, Sato M. 2004. Clinical features of sensitization to methamphetamine. *Ann. N.Y. Acad. Sci*. 1025:279–287.

Wang Z, Woolverton WL. 2007. Estimating the relative reinforcing strength of (+/-)-3,4-methylenedioxymethamphetamine (MDMA) and its isomers in rhesus monkeys:comparison to (+)-methamphetamine. *Psychopharmacology (Berl)*. 189:483–488.

Wu P, Liu X, Pham TH, Jin J, Fan B, Jin Z. 2010. Ecstasy use among US adolescents from 1999–2008. *Drug Alcohol Depend*. 142:33–38.

Yamamoto B, Moszczynska A, Gudelsky GA. 2010. Amphetamine toxicities: classical and emerging mechanisms. *Ann. N.Y. Acad. Sci.* 1187:101–121.

4

Cocaine

Learning Objectives

The student will learn:

1. What is the mechanism of action of cocaine?
2. What are the central effects of cocaine?
3. What are the peripheral effects of cocaine?
4. The effects of crack cocaine on drug use.
5. What is cross reinstatement?
6. The receptors involved in reinstatement of cocaine use.

Cocaine is found in the leaves of the South American coca bush, *Erythroxylum coca*. The natives of Peru have used the leaves of this bush for many hundreds of years for the stimulant effect produced when the leaves are chewed. The natives used the leaves primarily to improve their ability to work at high altitudes without becoming fatigued.

Considerable mystical significance was attributed to the coca leaf and to the powers of cocaine, because it enhanced the depressed human spirit. It was used in religious ceremonies in Peru, but eventually was also used as a form of money, shortly before the conquest by Spain. The Spanish continued this custom of using the coca leaf as payment for work in the gold and silver mines (See the structural formula for cocaine, Figure 4.1).

The history of cocaine is a long and colorful one. However, the Europeans did not accept cocaine, obtained from the coca leaf, until the middle of the nineteenth century. A French chemist, A. Mariani, was probably the most influential in bringing the coca leaf extract to the attention of Europe. He imported the coca leaves, extracted them and added this extract to wine, and called it "Coca Vin," for the fatigue of mind and body. Coca wine became so popular that even the Pope presented a medal of appreciation to Mariani (Karch, 2002).

The leaves of the coca bush contained not only the oils from the leaf but also the active chemical cocaine. Approximately 2% can be extracted as

---

Drugs of Abuse: Pharmacology and Molecular Mechanisms, First Edition. Sherrel G. Howard.
© 2014 John Wiley & Sons, Inc. Published 2014 by John Wiley & Sons, Inc.

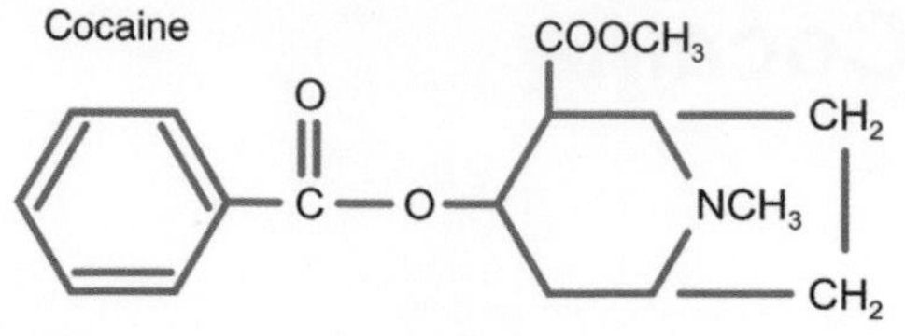

Figure 4.1   Structural formula for cocaine.

cocaine from the coca leaf. Once a constant supply could be guaranteed, cocaine became more interesting to the medical community. Freud wrote that it (cocaine) was a "magical drug" and he felt it would be useful as a safe exhilarant in his patients. More importantly Freud recommended cocaine as a safe drug, which eliminated the cravings from morphine withdrawal.

Karl Koller, an ophthalmologist and friend of Freud, examined the local anesthetic properties of cocaine and used cocaine during ophthalmic surgery. Today, cocaine or analogs of cocaine could still be used in ophthalmic and dental surgery as a local anesthetic. However, due to the abuse potential, cocaine's use is limited.

MECHANISM OF ACTION

Cocaine inhibits Uptake I, thereby blocking the reuptake of dopamine (DA), norepinephrine (NE), and serotonin (5-HT) that has been released into the synaptic cleft (See Figure 4.2). Cocaine does not directly stimulate the receptor normally activated by any of the monoamines, but acts by inhibiting the removal of the neurotransmitter from the synaptic cleft by blocking reuptake. Cocaine forms a complex with the DA transporter protein, as well as with NE transporter and the 5-HT transporter (SERT), thus blocking the transporter's ability to remove the monoamines from the synaptic cleft.

Cocaine has a similar effect on 5-HT, increasing the stimulation of particularly 5-HT2 and 5-HT3 receptors. While it is unclear as to what role 5-HT plays in the abuse of cocaine, 5-HT does seem to contribute to its overall effect.

The affinity for the dopamine transporter protein (DAT) is not the cause of the pronounced effect on DA reuptake. Recent research suggests that cocaine binds to the DAT in such a way as to produce a conformational change (Beuming et al., 2008). The binding of cocaine to the DAT actually stabilizes the transporter. This conformational change of the transporter is not seen with amphetamine or its analogs.

Cocaine is classified as a psychomotor stimulant or as an indirectly acting sympathomimetic.

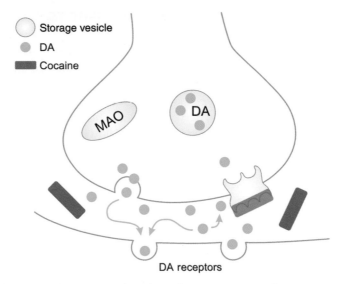

Figure 4.2   Cocaine blockade of the dopamine transporter protein.

Chronic cocaine use stimulates the mesocorticolimbic DA neurons in the ventral tegmental area (VTA) that terminate in the nucleus accumbens and the prefrontal cortex. According to several studies, this will lead to stimulation of the glutamatergic system and may constitute a "reward center" (Liuch et al., 2005; Kalivas et al., 2009).

Cocaine is also an agonist at sigma receptors and blocks Na+ channels. However, the inhibition of monoamine reuptake is considered to be the primary mechanism of action.

CENTRAL NERVOUS SYSTEM EFFECTS

Cocaine acts as an uptake inhibitor and a local anesthetic. As a local anesthetic, its primary clinical action lies in its ability to block the initiation or conduction of nerve impulses both centrally and in the periphery.

The effects of cocaine in the central nervous system (CNS) are similar to amphetamine, among the central effects of cocaine are as follows.

1. Produces euphoria or excitement.
2. Magnification of pleasurable experiences.

With prolonged use or excessive binging, paranoid delusions, hallucinations, tachycardia, and akathisia, which are all common to amphetamine abuse, will occasionally occur with cocaine abuse. As tolerance develops and the dose of cocaine is increased by the user, the side effects are tremors and with increasing dosage convulsions. These are followed by respiratory depression and vasomotor depression.

PERIPHERAL NERVOUS SYSTEM EFFECTS

In the peripheral nervous system, cocaine acts as a local anesthetic, blocking nerve conductance, thus potentially altering the functioning of all organ systems, muscle fibers, autonomic ganglia, and the neuromuscular junction. Cocaine also acts by inhibiting monoamine uptake or reuptake in the peripheral nervous system. This action produces an increase in sympathetic activity leading to the following.

1. Tachycardia
2. Increase in blood pressure
3. Increase in cardiac output
4. Vasoconstriction
5. Body temperature may increase (due to increased motor activity coupled with reduced heat loss from the vasoconstriction)

This action is called a *sympathomimetic effect* in that it mimics the effect of stimulating the sympathetic nervous system.

CHRONIC USE OF COCAINE

The chronic use of cocaine produces a downregulation of both DA and 5-HT receptors. There is a reduction in the concentration of DA and 5-HT in the brain, resulting in a dysphoria/depression that is felt after the initial high. The side effects from continued use can range from chest pain, asthma, shortness of breath and a general flu-like syndrome. Chronic "snorting" of cocaine causes degradation of the nasal septum and eventual disappearance. Chronic use increases the risk of hemorrhagic and ischemic strokes.

Toxic effects occur commonly in chronic cocaine users. The primary acute dangers are

1. Cardiac arrhythmias
2. Coronary thrombosis
3. Cerebral thrombosis
4. Heart failure (due to damage to the myocardium)

PHYSICAL DEPENDENCE AND WITHDRAWAL

Like amphetamine, cocaine does not produce a severe physical withdrawal syndrome, but rather produces depression on withdrawal of the drug, creating a drug craving to stop the depression. Withdrawal of cocaine also produces a marked deterioration of motor performance and learned behavior, vivid dreams or nightmares, insomnia increased appetite and irritability.

While cocaine produces no pronounced physical dependence, there is an enormous psychological dependence formed. The pattern of occasional use and escalating dosage is soon followed by compulsive binges. This pattern is identical to that seen with amphetamine.

PHARMACOKINETICS

Cocaine is easily absorbed by a variety of routes of administration. For many years the most common form of cocaine was the hydrochloride salt, which could be administered either by nasal inhalation or by intravenous injection. The intravenous route of administration produces an intense and immediate euphoria and the duration of action is roughly 30–60 minutes. This is a much shorter duration of action than that seen with amphetamine. Nasal inhalation produces a less dramatic high and also tends to cause atrophy and necrosis of the nasal mucosa and nasal septum.

There was a dramatic increase in the use of cocaine when the free base form (crack cocaine) became available as a street drug. Unlike the hydrochloride salt, crack cocaine could be smoked. Crack cocaine produces a rapid and intense effect, with less risk from contaminated needles, which could occur with the intravenous route or the danger of atrophy or necrosis of the nasal mucosa, which might be produced by the inhalation route of administration. The ramifications of this drug becoming cheap and readily available produced far-reaching social and economic consequences.

METABOLISM

While there are many metabolites or breakdown products of cocaine, the two primary metabolites are benzoylecgonine (BE) and methylecgonine ester (MEE). After ingestion, roughly 30–40% of the ingested cocaine can be found in the urine as BE. Similarly, 30–50% of the ingested cocaine can be measured in the urine as the metabolite MEE. Hospitals or clinics rarely measure any metabolite other than BE as it is found in the highest concentration and therefore easier to measure. Very little if any cocaine is found unmetabolized in the urine (Karch, 2002). Other studies have found that the concentrations of the metabolites vary considerably, with BE constituting roughly 80–90% of the cocaine administered (Jatlow, 1988). As methods for measuring the metabolites of cocaine have improved and become more sensitive, smaller amounts of the compounds can be analyzed. Metabolites of cocaine can now be measured in hair such that ones pattern of cocaine consumption can actually be monitored. These more sensitive assays have provided data demonstrating that the use of cocaine is much higher than previously suspected.

Tolerance

Tolerance develops fairly rapidly to the indirectly acting sympathomimetic drugs. Repeated doses of cocaine, which are necessary to produce the continued "high," eventually produce smaller and smaller central effects. A marked tolerance to the central effects develops with the repeated dosages, as in the binge situation, and accounts for the abuse liability of cocaine.

NEUROBIOLOGY OF RELAPSE

Cocaine Use or Cocaine Seeking

There are high rates of relapse to drug use following even prolonged withdrawal periods from cocaine or heroin use. Numerous studies examining the causes for cocaine or heroin relapse have been published (for a review see Shalev et al., 2002). Reinstatement models have been developed examining the primary causes for reinstatement, or to define the "triggers" that precipitate return to drug use. There are four different reinstatement models that have been extensively studied, individually or in combination. The "reinstatement model" is defined as resuming or returning to a previously conditioned response. In cocaine or heroin free individuals, drug craving and relapse to drug use can be triggered by:

1. Exposure to self-administered drug (drug priming);
2. Stimuli that are associated with drug taking (cues);
3. Exposure to multiple stressors;
4. Other neurotransmitter systems.

In animal experiments, after withdrawal from cocaine or heroin, cocaine seeking followed an inverted U-shaped curve. Cocaine seeking after exposure to previous cues remained elevated for at least 3 months, and finally starts to decrease after 6 months.

Drug Priming

Incubation of reward craving is not drug specific. Sugar (sucrose) seeking induced by re-exposure to the reward cues also increases after withdrawal, only for a shorter period of time.

Incubation of cocaine craving is not evident after an acute re-exposure to cocaine (drug priming). It is encouraging to know that cocaine seeking induced by cocaine priming remains unchanged over the first 6 months of withdrawal.

Neurotransmitters Involved

DA receptors are critically involved in cocaine reinstatement.

1. DA D_1 and D_2 receptors play different role.
2. Activation of DA D_2 receptor increases cocaine seeking.
3. Activation of DA D_1 receptor inhibits cocaine seeking.
4. Activation of $GABA_B$ or $5\text{-}HT_{2C}$ attenuates cocaine reinstatement.
5. Cannabinoids may also be involved in cocaine reinstatement.

Stress-Induced Reinstatement

Involvement in a single stressor does not seem to initiate cocaine-seeking behavior. However, exposure to several stressors does initiate cocaine-seeking behavior, and multiple stressors also have been shown to activate the mesocorticolimbic DA system.

It has long been accepted that the mesocorticolimbic DA system contributes to the acute reinforcing effects of cocaine. Cocaine is an indirect DA agonist and increases the concentration of DA extraneuronally by blocking the DA transporter and the reuptake of DA. Reinstatement of cocaine-seeking behavior has been examined in several ways:

1. Cocaine priming: cocaine is not necessary to produce reinstatement. Other drugs can produce "crossover generalization."

    Amphetamine is a very effective drug with which to prime the system. Drugs that "mimic" the effect of cocaine, that is, that produce similar behavioral or central effects, can induce crossover generalization. In fact, sugar is a weak primer for cocaine reinstatement.
2. DA D_1 agonists, which rats and monkeys will self-administer, block reinstatement.
3. DA D_2 antagonists attenuate reinstatement.

In summary, activation of DA D_2-like receptor agonists activate cocaine-seeking behavior, and activation of DA D_1-like receptor agonist will block reinstatement behavior.

Drugs even as innocuous as coffee (caffeine) have been shown to activate drug-seeking behavior. However, the response to caffeine may be due to an interaction between adenosine A_{2A} and the D_2 receptor, which are negatively coupled.

Blocking the adenosine A_{2A} receptor activates the DA D_2 receptor and cocaine-seeking behavior.

CROSS REINSTATEMENT

Cross reinstatement by a drug other than the initial self-administered drug is most commonly observed within a given drug class. See below for examples of drug groups.

Amphetamines	X	Cocaine
Barbiturates	X	Sedative hypnotics
Heroin	X	Morphine, methadone

While this paradigm for cross reinstatement of a drug generally holds true, there are exceptions. Stimulants can reinstate opioid-seeking behavior; however, opioids do not reinstate stimulant (i.e., amphetamine) seeking behavior.

GLUTAMATE AND REINSTATEMENT

Glutamate is one of the most ubiquitous transmitters in the brain, but has only recently been implicated in the formation of addiction as well as the reinstatement of addiction (Kalivas and O'Brien, 2008; Kalivas, 2009; Kalivas et al., 2009). Glutamate was implicated in the late 1990s as potentially being involved in the formation of drug addiction, when behavioral sensitization and motor stimulant effects were linked to glutamate, and it was determined that behavioral sensitization could be blocked with an antagonists of the NMDA subtype of the glutamate receptor. Over the past 10 years, an enormous amount of research has confirmed these initial findings and taken the research one-step further. It may, in the future, be possible to treat drug addiction with drugs specifically designed to block the NMDA receptor, thus reducing drug seeking and even possibly drug craving.

While the "reinstatement models" have been developed in non-human primates and rodents, they may not replicate the situations experienced by humans that lead to drug use or drug abstinence. It has been suggested by Bergman and Katz (1998) that the "reinforcement models" may not be an accurate model of relapse in humans. Nonetheless, many laboratories have used these models and studied the potential triggers that can precipitate drug relapse, and it can be stated that at least the models are predictive.

There is a common denominator between the four reinstatement models, namely that the mesocorticolimbic DA system is involved in compulsive drug use. The effects of the drug on the brain, rather than the withdrawal of the drug, may be the critical factor in compulsive drug use and/or relapse (Shalev et al., 2002). Shalev and coworkers summarized their finding by pointing out that a solution to drug relapse may only be found in a combination of pharmacological therapies, combining drugs that will attenuate stress-induced relapse with drugs that are effective against the abused drug or drug cues.

Review Questions

1. How are the withdrawal effects from cocaine the same, or different from the withdrawal effects from amphetamine or an analog of amphetamine?
2. What difference did the introduction of crack cocaine have on the use of cocaine?
3. Discuss the rate of relapse in cocaine use.
4. Which neurotransmitters are involved in the reinstatement of cocaine use?
5. Discuss stress-induced reinstatement.

REFERENCES AND ADDITIONAL READING

Beuming T, Kniazeff J, Bergmann ML, et al. 2008. The binding sites for cocaine and dopamine in the dopamine transporter overlap. *Nat. Neurosci.* 11:780–789.

Bossert JM, Gray SM, Lu L, Shaham Y. 2006. Activation of group II metabotropic glutamate receptors in the nucleus accumbens shell attenuates context-induced relapse to heroin seeking. *Neuropsychopharmacology.* 31:2197–2209.

Gipson CD, Reissner KJ, Kupchik YM, et al. 2013. Reinstatement of nicotine seeking is mediated by glutamatergic plasticity. *Proc. Natl Acad. Sci.* 110:9124–9129.

Jatlow P. 1988. Cocaine: analysis, pharmacokinetics and metabolic disposition. *Yale J. Biol. Med.* 61:105–113.

Kalivas PW. 2009. The glutamate homeostasis hypothesis of addiction. *Nat. Rev. Neurosci.* 10:561–772.

Kalivas PW, O'Brien C. 2008. Drug addiction as a pathology of staged neuroplasticity. *Neuropsychopharmacol. Rev.* 33:166–180.

Kalivas PW, Volkow ND. 2011. New medications for drug addiction hiding in glutamatergic neuroplasticity. *Mol. Psychiatry.* 16:974–986.

Kalivas PW, LaLumiere R, Knacksedt L, Shen H. 2009. Glutamate transmission in addiction. *Neuropharmacology.* 56:169–173.

Karch SB. 2002. *Karch's Pathology of Drug Abuse.* CRC Press, New York.

Liuch J, Rodriguez-Arias M, Aguilar MA, Minarro J. 2005. The role of dopamine and glutamate receptors in cocaine-induced social effects in isolated and grouped male OF1 mice. *Pharmacol. Biochem. Behav.* 82:478–487.

McFarland K, Kalivas PW. 2001. The circuitry mediating cocaine-induced reinstatement of drug-seeking behavior. *J. Neurosci.* 21:8655–8663.

Pickens CL, Airavaara M, Theberge G, Fanous S, Hope BT, Shaham Y. 2011. Neurobiology of the incubation of drug craving. *Trends Neurosci.* 34:411–420.

Shalev U, Grimm JW, Shaham Y. 2002. Neurobiology of relapse to heroin and cocaine seeking: a review. *Pharmacol. Rev.* 54:1–42.

Sun W, Akins CK, Mattingly AE, Rebec GV. 2005. Ionotropic glutamate receptors in the ventral tegmental area regulate cocaine-seeking behavior in rats. *Neuropsychopharmacology.* 30:2073–2081.

Xie X, Lasseter HC, Ramirez DR, Ponds KL, Wells AM, Fuchs RA. 2012. Subregion-specific role of glutamate receptors in the nucleus accumbens on drug context-induced reinstatement of cocaine-seeking behavior in rats. *Addiction Biol.* 17:287–299.

Part II Depressants, Sedative Hypnotics, and Anxiolytics

5 Benzodiazepines and Barbiturates

Learning Objectives

The student will learn:

1. The mechanism of action of the benzodiazepines and the barbiturates.
2. The central effects of the benzodiazepines and the barbiturates.
3. What is the primary difference between an anxiolytic and a sedative-hypnotic?
4. To recognize the symptoms of dependency and withdrawal from benzodiazepines.
5. How pharmacokinetics play a role in determining the severity of the withdrawal symptoms.

Librium was first synthesized in 1961 at the Hoffman La Roche laboratories. The synthesis was actually brought about by a laboratory accident. After the accident, tests revealed a compound with a seven-sided ring was created during the explosion and they decided to test it.

Prior to the discovery of librium, barbiturates like pentobarbital (Nembutal), or secobarbital were used to reduce both emotional and skeletal muscle tension, while phenobarbital was used to treat chronic conditions and in fact the barbiturates are still very useful. However, it was recognized that dependence on barbiturates was easily formed. This led to the search for a newer class of drugs, ones that would act as a muscle relaxant, anti-anxiety or sleep-inducing drug and not prove as addicting (Figure 5.1).

The characteristics of the anxiolytics and the sedative hypnotics are very similar. In many cases, it will seem as though we are discussing them almost interchangeably. This is because one can take an anxiolytic and by increasing the dose have a sedative hypnotic (Figure 5.1).

Drugs of Abuse: Pharmacology and Molecular Mechanisms, First Edition. Sherrel G. Howard.
© 2014 John Wiley & Sons, Inc. Published 2014 by John Wiley & Sons, Inc.

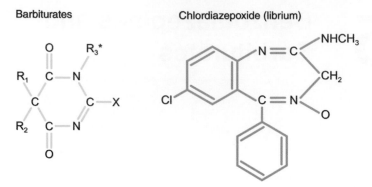

Barbiturates   Chlordiazepoxide (librium)

Figure 5.1   General structure for barbiturates.

The benzodiazepines fall into two categories as follows.

1. Anxiolytic—These are drugs used to treat anxiety.
2. Hypnotic (sedative hypnotic)—These are drugs used to treat insomnia.

Even though the clinical objectives are different, the same drugs are often used for both purposes. This is a reflection of the fact that drugs that treat anxiety generally cause some degree of sedation or drowsiness. The drowsiness is one of the main drawbacks in the clinical use of anxiolytic drugs. In high doses, the benzodiazepines and the barbiturates can produce unconsciousness, and the barbiturates can potentially result in death from respiratory and/or cardiovascular depression. There are many new drugs in the class of compounds called benzodiazepines now on the market. However, it should be remembered that all of these drugs produce drug dependence.

Several factors are used to determine whether a drug is used to treat anxiety or insomnia. The critical factor that is considered is the slope of the dose–response curve for central nervous system (CNS) depression. A sedative with a very shallow dose–response curve can be used to treat anxiety because there is a wide dose range available to produce the desired calming effect without the undesirable side effects such as drowsiness, ataxia, and slurred speech. A sedative with a steep dose–response curve will be used to treat insomnia. The ideal sedative hypnotic would be rapidly absorbed, producing drowsiness quickly, and then be rapidly metabolized and excreted, such that when you wake in the morning you do not have that "groggy" feeling.

We are all familiar with Ambien or Halcion. These are short-acting drugs, which rapidly induce sleep (Figure 5.2). However, one of the first drugs in this category was meprobamate. It is similar to phenobarbital, but shorter acting. Meprobamate was used as an anxiolytic and a

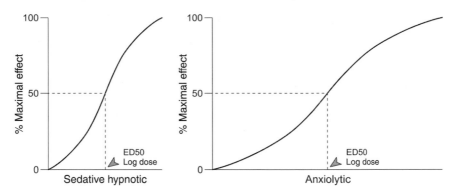

Figure 5.2   An example of a dose–response curve for an anxiolytic and a sedative hypnotic.

sedative hypnotic, but it produced the "groggy" morning feeling that was not wanted.

If we look at the pharmacokinetics of meprobamate, it is immediately obvious why newer, short-acting drugs were needed. Meprobamate is readily absorbed, but does not reach peak blood concentration for 1–2 hours after administration. Levels, or the concentration of meprobamate in the blood, then decline over a period of approximately 10 hours. This accounts for the "groggy" feeling experienced after taking meprobamate. Most of the meprobamate is excreted in urine within 24 hours, approximately 50% is excreted unchanged and some remaining meprobamate is hydroxylated. Hydroxymeprobamate has no activity. A sedative hypnotic that lasts for 10–12 hours is obviously not the sleep-inducing pill one wants to take when getting on an airplane. Even a 6–8 hour flight will not be long enough. Similarly, very few of us want to sleep for 10–12 hours every night.

MECHANISM OF ACTION

It was once thought that the benzodiazepines had a rather nonspecific mechanism of action. This was followed by a period of receptor-binding studies, where it was thought that there was a specific benzodiazepine receptor. We now know that the benzodiazepines act very selectively on the $GABA_A$ receptor, which mediates the fast inhibitory synaptic potential produced by activity in GABAergic neurons.

Benzodiazepines produce their effect by enhancing the response of the receptor to γ-aminobutyric acid (GABA). This is accomplished by facilitating the opening of the GABA-activated chloride channels (See insert in Figure 5.4). The benzodiazepines are binding to a regulatory site, not the receptor. The benzodiazepines act allosterically at this site to increase the

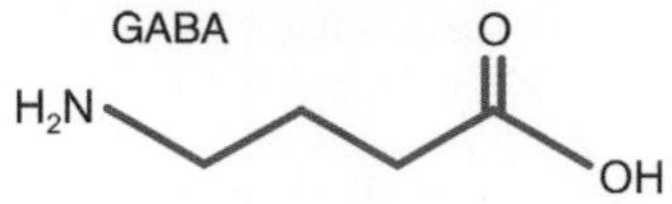

Figure 5.3   Structure of γ-aminobutyric acid (GABA).

affinity of GABA to the receptor. The powerful inhibitory effect of GABA on neurons was first discovered in the 1950s and its role as a neurotransmitter was hypothesized.

The mechanism of action of the benzodiazepines is very different from that of the barbiturates. GABA is known to initiate the fast inhibitory synaptic response. The effect of the benzodiazepines is to enhance the response of the receptor to GABA by facilitating the opening of the GABA-activated chloride channel. Benzodiazepines bind to a regulatory site, not the receptor, as was thought for so many years.

The benzodiazepines bind, with a very high affinity to the macromolecule that functions as the benzodiazepine receptor. $GABA_A$ receptors are the target for benzodiazepine and barbiturates. The benzodiazepines have a sedative and anxiolytic effect and selectively enhance the effect of GABA on $GABA_A$ receptors.

It seemed inconceivable that such simple compounds as the amino acids could actually be neurotransmitters (See Figure 5.3). However, a small group of scientists believed that some amino acids were more than just precursors. In Scotland, studies examining the role of glutamate as a neurotransmitter were being reported. When one amino acid (glycine) was finally established as an inhibitory neurotransmitter, the rest of the potential amino acid neurotransmitters followed quite rapidly.

To put these findings into perspective, the 1950s and 1960s might be considered as "prehistory," with respect to amino acid research, much akin to the Stone Age and the Dark Ages, respectively. During this time GABA was thought to be nothing more than a pharmacological curiosity. Continuing with this analogy, the 1970s would then be considered the Renaissance for amino acid research.

GABA is synthesized from glutamate by the enzyme glutamic acid decarboxylase (see Chapter 2). Much like the catecholamines, its action is terminated by reuptake, into the nerve ending, or deamination.

The group of drugs termed "anxiolytics" is divided into several groups, based primarily on their site of action. As can be seen in Table 5.1, not all anxiolytics act on the GABA receptor.

There have been thousands of benzodiazepines synthesized and roughly 20 or so are on the market today. They are basically similar in their pharmacological actions. The benzodiazepines have a broad spectrum of activity both centrally and peripherally. The effect of any specific benzodiazepine may be greater or more pronounced in one of the areas listed below with only a negligible effect in other areas.

Table 5.1   Classes of Anxiolytic Drugs

1. Benzodiazepines—The most important drug in this group.
2. Serotonin 1A receptor agonists—These are anxiolytics that produce very little sedation.
3. Barbiturates—Anxiolytic and sedative.
4. β adrenoceptor antagonists—Primarily reduces physical symptoms.
5. Miscellaneous drugs.

Benzodiazepines do not have antidepressant activity as a rule. The benzodiazepines, however, do produce a response in some people that is called a 'PARADOXICAL EFFECT." In this small group of people the benzodiazepines produce irritability and aggression. These symptoms may be particularly pronounced with some of the ultrashort-acting compounds, but can also be seen with valium and librium. The response may be due to a withdrawal syndrome, which would be more pronounced in the ultrashort-acting compounds.

PHYSICAL DEPENDENCE

Dependence to Ambien or Halcion can develop fairly rapidly. After several days of use, the seizure threshold starts to be reduced. After 2 weeks, the seizure threshold is below normal and withdrawal hyper-excitability can be detected within 4–8 hours after the last dose was taken.

Today, anxiolytic drugs are the most frequently prescribed drugs in this country. It is sometimes easier to prescribe an anxiolytic than to talk to the patient for a short time (Table 5.2). Anxiolytics are prescribed to treat anxiety, which can include phobic anxiety and/or panic disorder. The distinction between these and generalized anxiety is not a sharp line and the anxiolytic drugs are used to treat all of them.

WITHDRAWAL FROM BENZODIAZEPINES

There were early claims that benzodiazepines did not produce dependence. This is not true and while it posed a major problem at the time, it is now recognized that dependence can be produced even when therapeutic doses are used.

Table 5.2   Pharmacological Effects of Benzodiazepines

Decrease anxiety and aggression
Sedation, i.e., sleep producing
Decreased muscle tone
Anti-convulsant activity

SYMPTOMS OF WITHDRAWAL FROM BENZODIAZEPINES

Increased anxiety
Tremor
Dizziness
Early morning insomnia

The withdrawal symptoms produced when stopping benzodiazepine treatment are slower in onset and less intense than those found from barbiturate withdrawal. This may be due to the long half-life of some of the benzodiazepines, or alterations that may have occurred at the level of the receptor. In support of the correlation between withdrawal symptoms and half-life, shorter-acting benzodiazepines produce more abrupt withdrawal symptoms than the longer-acting benzodiazepines.

Conditions That Alter Duration and Intensity of Withdrawal

The conditions necessary to develop dependency have been extensively examined, as well as "what type of patient" will develop severe withdrawal symptoms when the medication is stopped. **Dose and duration** were among the first variables to be tested. Experiments were designed such that patients were treated with a lower dose of drug in a substitute form, so that they would not know the dose of their medication was reduced. These patients did develop an increase in cortisol levels and an increase in anxiety during the reduction and withdrawal period, which was greater than that for patients receiving their full dose of a benzodiazepine.

The effects on withdrawal, following termination of short-acting benzodiazepines were compared with withdrawal from the longer-acting benzodiazepines. Patients took the drug for 4 weeks and then the drug was abruptly withdrawn. Both groups of patients, Group 1, the short-acting drug and Group 2, the long-acting drug, showed an improvement in symptoms of anxiety. After the drug was withdrawn, some improvement was maintained. However, there was a temporary increase in anxiety on withdrawal, which increased over a 3-day period. After 7 days, patients on the longer-acting benzodiazepine had returned to pre-withdrawal anxiety levels, while those on the short-acting benzodiazepine still had an increase in their level of anxiety. In most cases, abrupt withdrawal of short-acting benzodiazepines produced a more severe withdrawal than abrupt withdrawal from a longer-acting benzodiazepine.

Duration

Duration of exposure has been examined, comparing withdrawal symptoms in patients taking short-acting benzodiazepines and those taking long-acting benzodiazepines. When you consider time as the only factor,

patients taking benzodiazepines for more than 5 years suffered more severe withdrawal symptoms than those taking the drug for a shorter period
of time. However, the short-acting benzodiazepines produced the most severe withdrawal symptoms after long-term treatment. This may be due to
stores of drug in the adipose tissue that would slowly leave the system.

Not all patients develop a physical dependence. So one must ask what
determines who will develop a physical dependence to a benzodiazepine.
While a variety of factors have been examined, only a few were demonstrated to have any effect on the withdrawal syndrome.

The variables that did produce a significant effect on the withdrawal
syndrome are the following.

1. Short versus long-acting benzodiazepines; this is probably due to stor-
    age of drug in adipose tissue.
2. Tapering the drug withdrawal does decrease the intensity of the with-
    drawal symptoms.

However, no matter how one dealt with the process of withdrawal, rebound insomnia occurred following discontinuation of drug.

Factors That Influence the Withdrawal Response

In studies examining gradual versus abrupt withdrawal of a benzodiazepine, as the tapering started in the gradual withdrawal group, it was
noted that new symptoms appeared. Patients reported an increase in fear,
anxiety, vision changes, muscle twitching, and confusion, all positive in-
dications of a withdrawal syndrome. It was concluded that even though
abrupt withdrawal from a benzodiazepine produced more severe withdrawal symptoms, they did not suffer from the fear and anxiety reported
by the gradual withdrawal group.

Factors That Influence Elimination

1. Decreased hepatic function in patients with liver disease will have an
    increase in the half-life of the drug.
2. Microsomal enzyme activity may be increased. Barbiturates and ben-
    zodiazepines induce (increase activity of) microsomal enzymes.

Benzodiazepines are less likely to change hepatic enzymes with chronic
use.

Long-Term Outcome

There are very favorable outcomes reported for patients completing a full
withdrawal program. These patients were also most successful at main-
taining abstinence. The studies that followed long-term abstinence found

that those patients that completed a withdrawal program, for either benzodiazepines or barbiturates, reported fewer problems with anxiety and depression than prior to drug therapy.

PHARMACOKINETICS

In treating anxiety or sleep disorders, the benzodiazepines are taken orally. The rate of absorption is important to know with these drugs since it will determine how quickly they will produce drowsiness or begin to reduce anxiety. This will depend on the pH in the stomach. Drugs like the barbiturates are lipid soluble, and they will get into the blood stream very rapidly. Weak bases, such as the benzodiazepines are absorbed at a higher pH, and therefore are usually absorbed from the duodenum, which is not as acidic as the stomach. The time required to pass into a less acidic area may also account for a slower onset of action. Benzodiazepines are not given intramuscularly (IM) as this route of administration does not produce reliable absorption.

Lipid solubility plays a major role in determining the speed in which a drug gets into the CNS.

Drugs go first to the following.

1. Highly perfused tissue, like skeletal muscle and lungs.
2. More slowly into adipose tissue.

These processes also contribute to their termination, where the rate of metabolic transformation and elimination is too slow to account for the time required for dissipation of pharmacological effects. Drugs that are highly lipid soluble can be stored in fatty tissue. When drugs are stored in fatty tissue it increases the length of time required for pharmacological effects to dissipate. A good example of this would be the half-life of librium, which is 24 hours. However, at higher doses the half-life is 48 hours.

Many of the benzodiazepines or sedative hypnotics are biotransformed to a water-soluble metabolite before being cleared from the body. This transformation occurs by microsomal enzyme systems in the liver. The elimination half-life of the individual drugs depends on the rate of metabolic transformation (Table 5.3). This can be highly variable and depends on a number of factors such as acidity of stomach, other drugs in the system using the same metabolic enzymes, time since last meal, etc.

The benzodiazepines, aside from the desired calming or sleep-inducing effects also produce some unwanted side effects. Of these side effects depression and daytime sedation are the most problematic. It is possible that

Table 5.3 Examples of Half-Life Times for
a Few Drugs in This Category

Hexabarbital	a few hours
Barbiturate	18–48 hours
Phenobarbital	4–5 days
Librium	5–30 hours/
	24–48 hours
Flurazepam	100 hours

Flurazepam forms an active metabolite that is
eliminated very slowly.

the long half-lives of some of these benzodiazepines are responsible for the
undesirable side effects.

Benzodiazepines are excreted, as water-soluble metabolites primarily
through the kidney and changes in renal function do not alter the elimination of these metabolites. In order to increase the rate of elimination,
it is necessary to increase the pH of the urine. Since the benzodiazepines
are weak bases, making the urine more alkaline will increase excretion of
these drugs.

TOXICITY

An acute overdose of a benzodiazepine is considerably less dangerous
than it is for other anxiolytic/sedative hypnotic drug. While these agents
are often used in attempted suicide, the advantage is that they are rarely
successful. Often the patient is simply allowed to "sleep it off." However,
if alcohol is present, this combination can produce respiratory depression,
which is life threatening. While an overdose can be counteracted with
drugs like flumazenil, this treatment is not without the risk of precipi-
tating a seizure. So the usual course of action would be to simply "wait
it out."

TOLERANCE AND DEPENDENCE

Tolerance can occur with all benzodiazepines, as can dependence. These
are two properties shared by the benzodiazepines and the barbiturates.
The development of tolerance to the benzodiazepine is less marked than
that found with the barbiturates. While a tolerance to many of the side
effects of the benzodiazepines does develop, a tolerance to the sleep-
inducing effect of the benzodiazepines does not seem to occur.

Benzodiazepines produce tolerance by producing changes at the level of the receptor.

Barbiturates produce tolerance by inducing hepatic enzymes.

BARBITURATES

The effects of the barbiturates and the benzodiazepines are seemingly very similar. However, the barbiturates are potentially far more dangerous. Tolerance develops easily and quickly to barbiturates. Tolerance to the sedative and hypnotic actions will develop within 2 weeks.

Tolerance is transferred from one barbiturate to another. This is an example of cross-tolerance (cross-tolerance is the ability to switch from one barbiturate to another with no withdrawal or alteration of effect). It is important to note, however, when a tolerance has developed, for example, to the sedative properties of a particular barbiturate, a normal sensitivity still remains to the lethal dose (tolerance to the lethal dose does not occur).

Barbiturates are unquestionably habit forming and persons who are used to taking one tablet at bedtime for sleep will find this habit difficult to give up and develop a craving for the drug. This craving for barbiturates and the applied term of addiction does meet the World Health Organization's definition of addiction and physical dependence. The timeline of the physiological responses to barbiturates can be found in Table 5.4.

Table 5.4   Time Line of Events for Chronic Use of Barbiturates

1. Begin using one dose as a hypnotic
2. Tolerance develops
3. Need higher dose for the same effect
4. Lethal dose has not changed

MECHANISM OF ACTION

The mechanism of action of barbiturates is thought to be similar to that of the benzodiazepines in that they modulate the $GABA_A$ receptors (Loscher and Rogawski, 2012). Barbiturates bind to the $GABA_A$ receptor at the β subunit, a site that is distinct from the GABA-binding site and also different from the benzodiazepine-binding site (Figure 5.4). While barbiturates potentiate the effect of GABA, they also block the AMPA receptor (AMPA receptors are a subtype of glutamate receptors). So taken together, barbiturates potentiate inhibitory $GABA_A$ receptors, as well as inhibit the excitatory AMPA receptor.

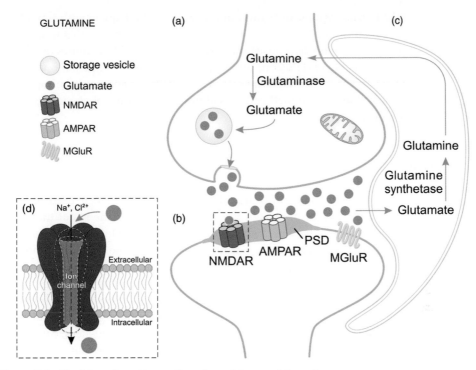

Figure 5.4   The interaction of benzodiazepines at the regulatory site.

ACUTE POISONING

Because of the widespread use of barbiturates as sedative hypnotics, there are ample opportunities for their involvement in accidental intoxication and/or suicide, particularly when taken with alcohol.

Treatment of barbiturate poisoning consists of the following.

1. Removing any undissolved drug from the stomach.
2. Support respiration.
3. Support cardiovascular system.
4. Increase elimination of drug by making urine more alkaline.
5. Can treat with a stimulant.

The progression of symptoms with increasing doses starts with hypotension, shock, cardiovascular collapse, and renal failure leading finally to death.

The severity of the abstinence syndrome depends on the individual and the dose and duration of drug use. Abrupt withdrawal from the chronically intoxicated patient should be avoided, as too rapid withdrawal will lead to convulsions and grand mal seizures. An adequate withdrawal period would range anywhere from 3–7 days long. During this time many patients develop psychoses that are preceded by 24–48 hours of insomnia, consisting of delusions and visual and auditory hallucinations. These psychoses may last anywhere from 3 days to 3 months. It is important to note that seizure medication will not stop seizures of abstinence from barbiturates.

ADDICTION

The treatment for barbiturate addiction is similar to that used for narcotic addiction, even though the withdrawal syndrome is not that similar. A characteristic withdrawal syndrome will develop if the doses used were large enough and the barbiturate or any of the sedative hypnotics were taken for an extended period of time. The withdrawal syndrome is not exactly like a narcotic withdrawal, but presents in a different manner. Initially the user appears to improve as signs of barbiturate intoxication wears off. After 10–15 hours of abstinence the signs of withdrawal begin. There is an increase in anxiety, insomnia, nervousness, cardiovascular irregularities, nausea, and vomiting. It is possible that convulsions or seizures will develop on the second or third day of abstinence. Following the seizures a characteristic psychosis develops, with agitation, insomnia, delusions, and possibly even hallucinations. The psychosis resembles that seen with alcohol withdrawal, and it is significantly different from the withdrawal seen with narcotics. This withdrawal is longer lasting than withdrawal from narcotics and potentially life threatening (Fraser et al. 1953).

USE IN THE ELDERLY OF BENZODIAZEPINES OR BARBITURATES

Physical dependence on benzodiazepines or barbiturates in the elderly is not only common, but of considerable concern. The number of prescriptions for benzodiazepines, in the elderly patient, accounts for a significant portion of benzodiazepine sales. The barbiturates were at one time the drug of choice in the treatment of anxiety or insomnia. While they have been largely replaced by the benzodiazepines, they are still often used because of the low cost. In the older patient, sleep disorders are more common as are certain types of anxiety. The diagnosis for their prescription is rarely stated and they obtain these prescriptions along with prescriptions for other disorders, never knowing why they are taking these drugs. This is then long-term use for no particular reason and it would be difficult to withdraw these patients from their sedative hypnotic medication because of the withdrawal symptoms they would experience. The elderly pose an additional problem in that they are less able to metabolize barbiturates, such that they are more likely to have problems with a drug overdose.

USE IN THE PREGNANT OR NURSING FEMALE

Pregnant women who are dependent on, either a benzodiazepine or a barbiturate will deliver a dependent baby. Benzodiazepines and barbiturates pass through the placental barrier and are taken up by the fetus. Thus women dependent on either group of drugs will deliver a baby that will exhibit a withdrawal syndrome of varying severity. The withdrawal syndrome is similar to that seen in heroin withdrawal in the newborn and usually the newborn is treated with a benzodiazepine to ease the symptoms.

Benzodiazepines and barbiturates will also diffuse into breast milk producing a very lethargic baby.

DISTRIBUTION IN THE CENTRAL NERVOUS SYSTEM

Numerous sites in the CNS have been identified as being sensitive to this group of drugs. However, if we consider how different they are structurally it is amazing that they all produce relatively the same behavioral response/effect.

Very low doses of these drugs produce changes in the above CNS areas, that is, depression of evoked potentials (Table 5.5).

PHARMACODYNAMICS OF SEDATION

Sedation produces a decrease in responsiveness. The sedative hypnotics induce sleep and they also interrupt the sleep cycle.

Table 5.5   Sites of Action for Barbiturates and Benzodiazepines

Barbiturates have sites of action in the following.

1. Midbrain reticular formation
2. Posterior hypothalamus
3. Amygdala
4. Limbic structures
5. Hippocampus

Benzodiazepines have sites of action in the following.

1. Limbic system
2. Thalamus
3. Midbrain reticular formation

The result of taking a sedative hypnotic is as follows.

Latency till onset of sleep decreases.
Duration of non-rapid eye movement (nREM) sleep increases.
Duration of rapid eye movement (REM) sleep decreases.

The importance of slow wave or REM sleep only began to be understood with the increase in use of anxiolytics or sleep-inducing drugs. To date there is no perfect sleep-inducing drug—except maybe warm milk and a banana.

Anesthesia

Sedative hypnotics at high doses will depress the CNS to the point of stage III of general anesthesia. This is not an adequate level for deep surgery; however, it is perfectly adequate for short surgeries.

Anticonvulsant

Most of the drugs in the three classes of drugs we have considered are capable of inhibiting the spread of epileptiform activity in the CNS. However, some are far more selective than others.

Examples of benzodiazepine or barbiturate used to treat epilepsy are the following.

Phenobarbital good
Diazepam good
Nitrazepam infantile spasm

EFFECT ON CARDIOVASCULAR AND RESPIRATORY SYSTEMS

Healthy patients will have almost "no change" in respiration after either a benzodiazepine or a barbiturate. Respiration will be at a rate very similar to sleep. However, any of these drugs can produce respiratory depression. Similarly, in a normal patient there is no change in the cardiovascular system. But they can produce congestive heart failure in the unhealthy patient. At toxic doses, or particularly if there is renal impairment, myocardial contraction, and vascular tone are decreased.

Tolerance develops to all three groups of drugs as well as a cross-tolerance within the group of sedative hypnotics, where the benzodiazepines will substitute for alcohol.

The abuse of agents in all of these groups can be defined in both psychological and physiological terms. While the psychological addiction may parallel simple neurotic behavior, something difficult to separate from the heavy coffee drinker, as the pattern becomes more compulsive, more serious complications can develop including physical dependence and tolerance.

Review Questions

1. Describe the role of GABA and the effect of the benzodiazepines.
2. What are the withdrawal symptoms of a sedative-hypnotic?
3. Describe the toxicity of the benzodiazepines.
4. How do benzodiazepines and barbiturates produce tolerance?

REFERENCES AND ADDITIONAL READING

Ashton CH. 1991. Protracted withdrawal syndromes from benzodiazepines. *J. Subst. Abuse Treat.* 8:19–28.

Bain KT. 2006. Management of chronic insomnia in elderly persons. *Am. J. Geriatr. Pharmacother.* 4:168–192.

Fraser HF, Shaver, MR, Maxwell ES, Isbell H. 1953. Death due to withdrawal of barbiturates. *Am. J. Int. Med.* 38:1319–1325.

Geller I, Seifter J. 1980. The effects of meprobamate, barbiturates, d-amphetamine and promazine on experimentally induced conflict. *Psychopharmacologia.* 1:482–492.

Johnston GA. 1996. GABA A receptor pharmacology. *Pharmacol. Ther.* 69:173–198.

Loscher W. Rogawski MA. 2012. How theories evolved concerning the mechanism of action of barbiturates. *Epilepsia.* 53:12–25.

Olsen RW, Betz H. 2006. GABA and glycine. In Siegel GJ, Albers RW, Brady S, Price DD (eds), *Basic Neurochemistry: Molecular, Cellular and Medical Aspects,* 7th edn. Elsevier, London, pp. 291–302.

Part III Dissociative Anesthetics

6 Phencyclidine and Ketamine

> ## Learning Objectives
>
> The student will learn:
>
> 1. The mechanism of action of phencyclidine (PCP) and ketamine?
> 2. The effect of PCP and ketamine on the central nervous.
> 3. The effect of PCP and ketamine on the peripheral nervous system.
> 4. To define an "open channel" blocker.

Phencyclidine (PCP) is classified as a psychotomimetic, a dissociative anesthetic, and a hallucinogen. Chemically, it is a synthetic aryl-cyclohexylamine (Figure 6.1). PCP was first developed in the 1950s as a surgical intravenous anesthetic. Unfortunately, during clinical trials it was found to produce delirium, hallucinations, and generally disoriented behavior post surgery. It was however, very effective in veterinary medicine, making animals tranquil and serene. The name Sernyl was derived based on the serene behavior noted in animal studies. By 1979 PCP was rescheduled to a Schedule III drug, so it could no longer be used in veterinary medicine. (A Schedule III drug in the United States meaning that the ownership and distribution of PCP for nonmedical reasons was illegal.)

Ketamine, an analog of PCP, is the most widely used anesthetic in the world (Figure 6.1); however, there are disadvantages to the anesthetic. Ketamine has multiple pharmacological effects, as a stimulant, depressant, and hallucinogen with anesthetic properties. While it has many of the advantages of PCP, it also exhibits a few of the negative side effects. Ketamine is also used in veterinary medicine and is an excellent intravenous anesthetic.

The illicit use of PCP started in the early 1960s on the West Coast. PCP was cheap and easy to synthesize and could easily be added to tobacco or marijuana for a more controllable high. This route of administration

Drugs of Abuse: Pharmacology and Molecular Mechanisms, First Edition. Sherrel G. Howard.
© 2014 John Wiley & Sons, Inc. Published 2014 by John Wiley & Sons, Inc.

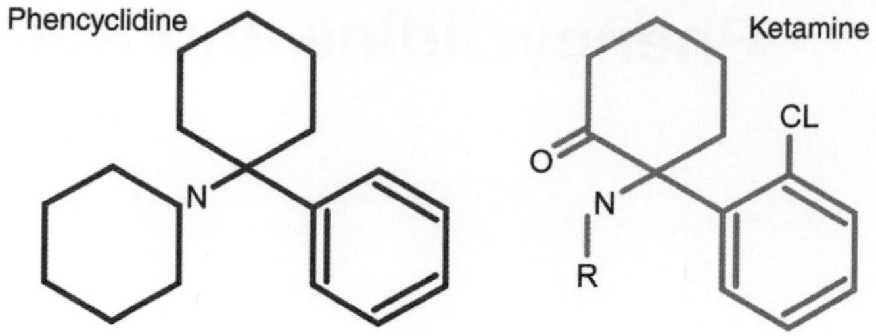

Figure 6.1   Structural formula of phencyclidine and ketamine.

tended to eliminate the "bad trip" or dysphoria that occurred after intravenous (IV) injection. To prevent the illegal synthesis of PCP, it was reclassified as a Schedule II drug, so that controls could be put on the precursor chemicals.

MECHANISM OF ACTION

PCP and ketamine act as noncompetitive antagonist of the NMDA subtype of glutamate receptors. It is "use dependent" in that it blocks an "open channel." While it is generally accepted that this is the primary mechanism of action of PCP and ketamine, there are other mechanisms that must also be considered. However, PCP also acts as an indirect dopaminergic agonist in some experimental models (Johnson and Jones, 1990). Interactions also occur with the noradrenergic and serotonergic neurotransmitter systems, but these interactions are poorly understood, and may not represent the primary mechanism of action of PCP or ketamine.

Ketamine and MK 801 are "open channel" blockers. While they exhibit many of the same properties as PCP, they do not have the same affinity for the receptor as PCP. The affinity of PCP for this site is ~0.2–1.0 uM, which just happens to be about the plasma concentration in humans when using PCP. PCP can also inhibit other channels, including:

1. Voltage dependent Na+ channels,
2. Potassium channels, and
3. ACh (The nicotinic receptor is also inhibited by PCP). ACh is inhibited by PCP in a non-competitive manner but is non-use dependent. PCP also acts on membrane proteins producing antagonism at the opioid receptor and the DA and NE transporter.

All of these effects of PCP are less potent than the effect on the NMDA receptor.

NEUROPHARMACOLOGY

Central Nervous System Effects of PCP or Ketamine

PCP produces a wide variety of effects in both humans and animals. In acute PCP intoxication, Gorelick and Balster (2002) cite three stages of PCP toxicity.

1. Behavioral toxicity
2. Stupor or light coma
3. Deep coma and unresponsiveness to pain

The most common behavior seen with PCP intoxication is delirium. Even in small doses PCP users experience euphoria and confusion, or lethargy and sedation. After using PCP, it is most common that there is an impairment of recent memory, disorientation, and possible impairment of judgment. Delirium can last for several days in PCP users when recovering from a light coma. Hallucinations are common, paranoid delusions, staring into space, and catalepsy are not uncommon.

PCP use has also been implicated in the bizarre and occasionally violent behavior seen in some drug users. Since PCP is an anesthetic, the PCP user can often cause severe damage to themselves or others. PCP does produce a feeling of invulnerability, and combined with impaired judgment has resulted in violent crimes or bizarre behavior. Common neurological effects are increased muscle tone, tremor, nystagmus, and ataxia (Gorelick and Balster, 2002).

Few drugs induce such a wide spectrum of effects, as does PCP (Table 6.1). It becomes easy to understand how a person using PCP can be misdiagnosed as schizophrenic as the two diseases have many presenting symptoms in common.

Peripheral Nervous System Effects of Phencyclidine or Ketamine

The effects on the PNS are varied, much like the CNS effects. Once again this may be due to dose, route of administration, or experience with the drug (Table 6.2). Pupil size may become enlarged or remain normal. Pupil size is reduced when the user goes into a coma.

The cardiovascular effects common to this group of drugs are due to sympathomimetic effects (stimulation of the peripheral sympathetic nervous system) and a decrease in baroreceptor stimulation. Usually one finds an elevation in heart rate and blood pressure, which will result in an increase in cardiac output.

Table 6.1   Effects of Phencyclidine at Different Dosages

Low dose	Euphoria	Sense of intoxication
	Staggering gait	Slurred speech
	Sweating	Numbness in extremities
	Muscle rigidity	Body image changes
	Drowsiness	Disorganized thought
	Apathy	Hostility
	Bizarre behavior	Delirium
Medium dose	Anesthesia	Analgesia more marked
	Stupor	Coma, but eyes are open
	Sweating	Sensory input distorted
	Fever	Increased heart rate and blood pressure
	Hyper salivation	Muscle rigidity
	Hallucinations	Delusions
High dose	Prolonged coma	Muscle rigidity
	Convulsions	
	On withdrawal of PCP: hallucinations, delirium, and anxiety	

Treatment will require a variety of drugs: neuroleptics for the resulting psychosis, sedative for anxiety and/or agitation, even Ca++ channel blockers have been used successfully.

CLINICAL USES FOR PHENCYCLIDINE AND KETAMINE

Ketamine was used as a battlefield anesthetic during the Vietnam Wars. Although it has fallen out of favor with the medical community due to the possibility of "emergence delirium" it is still occasionally used as an anesthetic with children and as an anesthetic in veterinary medicine (Domino,

Table 6.2   Peripheral Symptoms of Phencyclidine Depending on Dose

Average Dose of Phencyclidine
Sweating
Lacrimation (increase in tear formation)
Increased bronchial secretion
Increased saliva secretion
High Doses of Phencyclidine
Rhabdomyolysis (the break down of muscle tissue)
Acute renal failure (from myoglobinuria)
Apnea
Decreased heart rate
Hypotension (from decreased peripheral resistance)
Circulatory collapse
Seizures
Coma

2010). As a non-competitive antagonist of the NMDA receptors ketamine blocks transmission from the thalamus to the cortex, leading to the loss of ability to adequately interpret painful stimuli. Ketamine differs from many sedatives or anesthetics in that it maintains cardiovascular stability and spontaneous respiration, which made it a good battlefield anesthetic. It is also an excellent anesthetic in third world countries that do not have the resources to provide cardiovascular or respiratory stability. Ketamine is also effective in relieving chronic pain, neuropathic pain from phantom limb and pain resulting from cancer (Persson, 2013).

THE GLUTAMATE HYPOTHESIS OF SCHIZOPHRENIA

There are two different hypotheses as to the mechanisms underlying schizophrenia. The DA hypothesis attributes an increase in dopaminergic activity as the cause of schizophrenia, and the glutamate hypothesis attributes a decrease in glutamate activity as the underlying cause of schizophrenia. While there is ample evidence in favor of either hypothesis, the answer may lie somewhere in between. In fact the two hypotheses of schizophrenia compliment each other in that they reflect the complexity of the disease. Schizophrenia is diagnosed by examining the presence of positive symptoms (Type I symptoms) and negative symptoms (Type II symptoms). Positive symptoms are recognized by the presence of the symptom (Table 6.3), while negative symptoms are recognized as the absence of normal behavior.

The responses to PCP closely resemble many of the symptoms that are found in the schizophrenic patient. Most schizophrenic patients have both, positive, and negative symptoms or signs. Because the response to PCP also produces positive and negative signs, chronic PCP users are frequently misdiagnosed as having schizophrenia. Many drugs can produce hallucinations. However, PCP actually mirrors the symptoms

Table 6.3   Phencyclidine Induced "Positive" and "Negative" Signs of Schizophrenia

Positive Signs
1. Hallucinations (generally auditory or sensory; however, occasionally visual or olfactory)
2. Delusions
3. Thought insertion. You think someone else's thoughts are being put into your mind
4. Thought broadcasting. This is the belief that others can hear one's thoughts
5. Dysfunction of logical thought patterns

Negative Signs
1. Depression
2. Social withdrawal

Table 6.4   Comparison of Central Nervous System Markers in Schizophrenic Patients and Phencyclidine Users

Schizophrenic Patient	Phencyclidine User
Decrease in nicotinic receptors	Decrease in nicotinic receptors
Elevated dopamine in limbic area	Biphasic dopamine, but initially increased
Compromised K+ channel	Block K+ channel

of schizophrenia, and has been important in advancing research on this disease.

If we compare the clinical findings in schizophrenic patients with the effects of PCP we can further appreciate the similarities (Table 6.4).

It is clear that chronic low doses of PCP produce a pattern of metabolic and neurochemical changes that mirror the schizophrenic patient.

ROUTES OF ADMINISTRATION

PCP is easily synthesized and is found either in powder form or as a liquid. It is often contaminated with the precursor compounds used on the street, so the powder is not pure white in color. It is most commonly sprayed onto some leaf, such as marijuana, and then smoked. The free base form of pure PCP is a yellow oil, and this is often added to ether, and a cigarette can then be dipped in the liquid and smoked. The liquid was referred to as "embalming fluid" because it produced a somatic "numbing" effect combined with a feeling of dissociation. Unfortunately, users and dealers actually believe that the liquid PCP is made up of embalming fluid, and when PCP is in short supply, substitute embalming fluid for PCP.

CLINICAL USES

PCP was first tested shortly after World War II for use as an anesthetic in surgery. The adverse effects in humans, and the long half-life made it unsuitable for humans and it was marketed as a veterinary anesthetic. As it became a more popular street drug it was thought to be unsuitable for any medical use.

Ketamine is still used clinically as a short-acting dissociative anesthetic. It can be administered either IV or intramuscularly (IM) and within seconds it will begin to take affect. A sensation of numbness and dissociation occurs very rapidly. Amnesia and analgesia follow within 1 minute. After a single dose a patient will remain unconscious for approximately 10–15 minutes, additional doses may be used as needed. Ketamine is not recommended for most eye surgeries as intraocular pressure is increased. Since ketamine acts at the level of the cortex and limbic system, it takes several hours to awaken from a single anesthetic dose. Consciousness may be accompanied by hallucinations and "bad dreams."

ADDICTION AND ILLICIT USE OF PHENCYCLIDINE

It was thought that PCP did not lead to addiction. Drugs that simply alter perception, while not producing some type of reward or euphoria, like the dissociative anesthetics, were not considered to be addictive. This opinion has recently been challenged as animal studies have demonstrated that PCP does increase mesocorticolimbic dopamine concentrations, which can be rewarding. It could be argued that even if PCP did not produce addiction, it does produce a psychological dependence. The parallels between PCP intoxication and schizophrenia are so pronounced, that chronic use of PCP could lead to a schizophrenia-like psychosis that would be irreversible. Ketamine, while a weaker NMDA antagonist, also creates a psychological addiction. Tolerance to PCP and ketamine (Special K or Kit Kat) occurs fairly rapidly, with regular use. Frequent users of either drug must continually increase their dosage to obtain the same or similar high. Those users that inject PCP or ketamine and are chronic users, develop almost a permanent tolerance.

Death from ketamine overdose is rare, and despite its relative safety when used as an anesthetic it is not without side effects. The most common side effect is emergence delirium, and hallucinations. Some patients report that it may be comparable to a bad LSD trip (Persson, 2013). Other side effects include dizziness, blurred vision, nystagmus, nausea, vomiting, and tonic–clonic movements.

Withdrawal

The dependency produced by ketamine or PCP is a psychological dependence. Therefore the withdrawal does not produce the more severe withdrawal symptoms that drugs like the opioids produce. However, if the drug was associated with pleasurable experiences, then not having ketamine or PCP will produce an emotional withdrawal, depression, insomnia, and irritability. Drug cravings have been reported and even flashbacks do occur.

Effect on Performance

The effects on performance are primarily cognitive impairments. Distractibility is increased and hallucinations occur that are visual or sensory. Memory is significantly impaired, both recall and verbal language function is also impaired. In general, there is a decrease in awareness, lack of responsiveness, reaction time is increased and spatial perception is altered or distorted.

PHARMACOKINETICS

Distribution

PCP is rapidly cleared from blood and is taken up by the brain and easily penetrates into fatty tissue. The elimination of PCP from the body can take up to several weeks, as the stores of PCP are being slowly released from fatty tissue. As a lipophilic weak base, renal clearance of PCP is dependent on the pH of urine. The PCP binding sites at the NMDA receptor are widely distributed in human brain. The highest densities occur in the cerebellum, hippocampus, and temporal cortex (Weissman et al. 1991).

Metabolism

PCP is metabolized primarily by cytochrome P-450 dependent mixed function oxidases. This occurs in the liver. The majority of the administered dose (75%) is ring hydroxylated and excreted in urine. This pattern of PCP metabolism holds over a wide range of doses.

Ketamine is also metabolized by the P-450 system to norketamine and dehydronorketamine, which can be detected in urine (Okon, 2007).

Duration of Action

The onset of effects of PCP depends on the route of administration. If PCP is smoked or injected, then the onset of effects occurs very rapidly, within 1–2 minutes. The effects are somewhat delayed if PCP powder is snorted or taken orally, ~30 minutes. The duration of action (or the period of intoxication) may last for over 4–6 hours for a recreational dose. However, in some users the duration of action may be prolonged, lasting 24 hours and longer. Consciousness may return within an hour following an IV injection; however, the user may not return to "normal" for at least 24 hours. PCP may induce a psychotic reaction that could last more than 1 month. The half-life for elimination of PCP from plasma is 7–50 hour (mean 17.6 hour) (Gorelick and Balster, 2002).

The onset of action for ketamine also depends on the route of administration. When injected intramuscularly, the onset of effects occurs within 5 minutes and with a duration of action of approximately 30 minutes to 2 hours. Ketamine easily crosses the blood brain barrier and is also rapidly distributed thought out the body, going first to heart and lungs, then to muscle and finally being stored in adipose tissue (Haas, 1992). Ketamine elimination is primarily via the kidneys in the form of norketamine, with an elimination half-life of approximately 2 hours.

Review Questions

1. Compare the two different theories about the mechanism underlying schizophrenia.
2. What were the clinical uses for PCP and ketamine?
3. Describe the dependency produced by PCP and ketamine and the subsequent withdrawal symptoms.

REFERENCES AND ADDITIONAL READING

Domino EF. 2010. Taming the ketamine tiger. *Anesthesiology.* 113:678–686.

Gorelick David A, Balster Robert L. 2002. Phencyclidine (PCP). In: Davis KL, Charney D, Coyle JT, Nemeroff C (eds), *Neurophsychopharmacology: The Fifth Generation of Progress.* Lippincott Williams & Wilkins, Philadelphia.

Haas DA, Harper DG. 1992. Ketamine: a review of its pharmacologic properties and use in ambulatory anesthesia. *Anesth. Prog.* 39:61–68.

Johnson KM, Jones SM. 1990. Neuropharmacology of phencyclidine: basic mechanisms and therapeutic potential. *Annu. Rev. Pharmacol. Toxicol.* 30:707–750.

Okon T. 2007. Ketamine: An introduction for the pain and palliative medicine physician. *Pain Physician.* 10:493–500.

Persson J. 2013. Ketamine in pain management. *CNS Neurosci. Ther.* 19(6):1–7.

Weissman AD, Casanova MF, Kleinman JE, DeSouza EB. 1991. PCP and sigma receptors in brain are not altered after repeated exposure to PCP in humans. *Neuropsychopharmacology.* 258:207–215.

7

γ Hydroxybutyrate

Learning Objectives

The student will learn:

1. What is thought to be the mechanism of action of γ hydroxybutyrate (GHB).
2. The primary central nervous system (CNS) effects of GHB.
3. The primary peripheral nervous system effects of GHB.
4. What are some clinical uses for GHB?

γ hydroxybutyrate (GHB, sodium oxybate) is a four-carbon fatty acid (Figure 7.1). It was first synthesized in 1874, but it was not until 1960 that Laborit (Laborit, 1960) examined GHB for its potential use as a central nervous system (CNS) depressant or anesthetic in humans. Today, it is still used as an anesthetic in minor surgeries in some European countries, and as a treatment for narcolepsy in the United States. GHB is an interesting drug because it is not only an endogenous compound, it is used therapeutically, and it is also a drug of abuse.

MECHANISMS OF ACTION

GHB was synthesized as an analog of GABA that would be able to cross the blood–brain barrier (BBB). It is similar in its CNS depressant effects to the inhibitory neurotransmitter GABA; however, GHB can cross the BBB and GABA cannot. While the precise mechanism of action of GHB is not known, initial attempts at defining the action of GHB were made by comparing it to the mechanisms of action for GABA. GABAergic receptors do in fact account for part of the mechanism of action of GHB; however, other transmitter systems such as dopamine (DA), serotonin (5-HT),

Drugs of Abuse: Pharmacology and Molecular Mechanisms, First Edition. Sherrel G. Howard.
© 2014 John Wiley & Sons, Inc. Published 2014 by John Wiley & Sons, Inc.

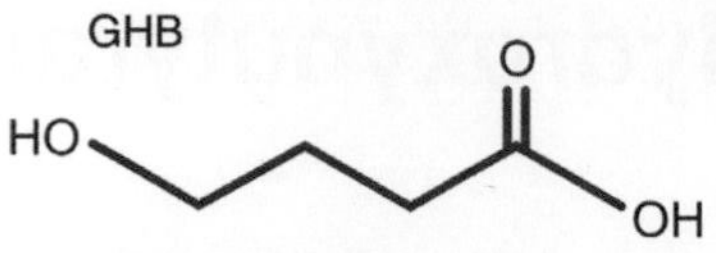

GHB

Figure 7.1   Chemical structure of γ hydroxybutyrate.

opioids, and a GHB-signaling system also account for some of the variety of effects produced by GHB.

GHB is found in many brain regions. Snead (1991) reported that the highest levels of GHB are found in the substantia nigra and in the ventral tegmental area. These areas have long been known to be rich in DA cell bodies (Dahlstrom and Fuxe, 1964). Since GHB is both a metabolite and a precursor of GABA (Figure 7.2), it is not surprising that it does share some common mechanisms of action with GABA.

EFFECTS OF γ HYDROXYBUTYRATE ON THE CENTRAL NERVOUS SYSTEM

Laborit examined the effects of GHB in humans describing the main central effects (Laborit, 1964). He found that GHB:

1. produces hypothermia
2. acts as a hypnotic
3. acts as an anesthetic
4. acts as an anti-convulsant

Of primary interest was the lack of respiratory depression that was found when anesthetic doses of GHB were used. The primary danger described by Laborit was the narrow therapeutic dose range. GHB was

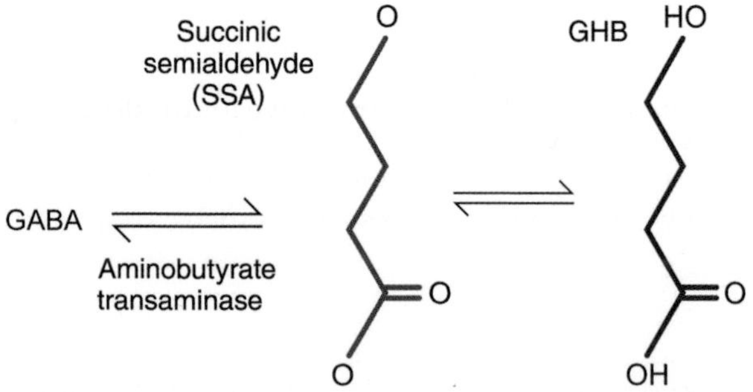

Figure 7.2   Synthesis and metabolism of γ hydroxybutyrate.

widely used in Europe as a hypnotic (to induce sleep), but was found to be dangerous when combined with alcohol or other CNS depressants.

γ HYDROXYBUTYRATE AND GABA RECEPTORS

There are two distinct binding sites for GHB in the CNS (Wu et al., 2004). While it has long been known that GHB binds to $GABA_B$ receptors, it has only recently been demonstrated that there is both a high- and low-affinity GHB-binding site, and that these binding sites have a very different distribution in the brain from that of the GABA receptors (Maitre, 1997; Crunelli et al., 2005). GHB is an agonist at the GHB receptor and exerts a stimulatory effect. At the $GABA_B$ receptor, it is a weak agonist, exerting an inhibitory effect at this receptor. GHB does not exhibit any significant degree of binding at the $GABA_A$ receptors.

Benavides and coworkers first identified the specific binding sites for GHB in 1982 (Benavides et al., 1982). The specificity of these receptor sites was based on the findings that baclofen did not displace tritium-labeled GHB (baclofen is a specific agonist at the $GABA_B$ receptor). Additionally, Snead (1994) demonstrated that GABA binding could not be detected until postnatal day 3, while labeled GHB binding was not observed until postnatal day 17. Taken together, these data provide compelling evidence for the existence of specific GHB receptor sites. Unfortunately, there are only a few selective compounds that act as specific ligands and aid in the determination of the role GHB receptors play or the functioning of the GHB-signaling system.

γ HYDROXYBUTYRATE AND DOPAMINE

There has been some controversy as to the role that GHB plays in modulating the neurotransmitter DA. The first pharmacological studies demonstrated that GHB had an inhibitory effect on DA. Some years later, using *in vivo* dialysis, it was demonstrated that GHB produced an increase in the release of DA, at low doses of GHB. The opposing studies fueled a controversy that continued for some years. What was not realized at this time was that GHB has a very steep dose–response curve (It was overlooked for many years that a narrow range for the dose–response curve was reported by Laborit in 1964.).

At low doses, GHB produces an increase in DA release.

At high doses, GHB produces a decrease in DA release.

The preponderance of evidence suggested that GHB inhibited DA release, which in turn activates tyrosine hydroxylase (TYOH) and thereby increases the concentration of DA in the brain by the following sequence of events.

1. It inhibits impulse flow in central DA neurons.
2. It stimulates synthesis of DA via negative feedback.
3. GHB increases intraneuronal DA levels.
4. GHB increases the levels of dihydroxyphenylacetic acid (DOPAC) in DA neurons.

The last three are a consequence of inhibiting impulse flow. Impulse flow is reduced in the mesolimbic DA system for over an hour. This would reduce/inhibit the release of DA. As a result, the concentration of DA in the synaptic cleft would be reduced. This reduction in the levels of DA will produce a negative feedback, which will in turn produce a disinhibition at presynaptic DA autoreceptors. This disinhibition produces an increase in intraneuronal DA synthesis. As a result of the increase in synthesis, DA levels increase within the terminals (the increased DA can be measured or visualized histologically). As DA starts to accumulate within the terminal, levels of the metabolite DOPAC also increase (Both DA and DOPAC can be measured using *in vivo* dialysis.). Howard and Banerjee (2002), attempting to bring together the various effects of GHB, while remaining consistent with known data put one possible hypothesis forth. These authors suggest a rather complex mechanism of action; they suggest that "GHB stimulates GHB receptors, or an isoform of the $GABA_B$ receptor, producing a decrease in the release of GABA. The resultant decrease in extracellular GABA would produce an increase in dopamine release at low doses and an inhibition of release of DA at higher doses, by K^+-dependent hyperpolarized cell membranes. Since the GHB receptors are on interneurons which contain both GABA and enkephalin, the interaction of these transmitters will also play a role in the final outcome" (Howard and Banerjee, 2002). This hypothesis does suggest that GHB is acting at a site that is separate from $GABA_B$ receptors and yet linked in some manner pre- or post-synaptically (Howard and Banerjee, 2002).

To date, there is only one compound, NCS-382, that is a specific antagonist of the GHB receptor. Unfortunately, the data obtained from electrophysiological studies using NCS-382 is difficult to interpret (Crunelli and Leresche, 2002).

THERAPEUTIC USES FOR γ HYDROXYBUTYRATE

γ *Hydroxybutyrate Use in the Treatment of Narcolepsy*

GHB became popular very quickly because it had few negative side effects and a short duration of action. Although the therapeutic dose range was very narrow, this was not initially viewed as a problem. It only became a problem when GHB was used in conjunction with other CNS depressants such as alcohol.

GHB has been approved to treat narcolepsy as well as daytime catalepsy, which can occur with narcolepsy. It is sold under the name of Xyrem (for review, see Fuller and Hornfeldt, 2003). Narcolepsy is a relatively rare condition, characterized by daytime sleepiness and an irresistible desire to sleep. There are other symptoms that occasionally accompany narcolepsy which are catalepsy, sleep paralysis, temperature changes, and loss of muscle tone.

The most common treatment for narcolepsy is a combination of a stimulant, such as amphetamine, ritalin or modafinil, and some drug to interrupt rapid eye-movement (REM) sleep, such as Xyrem (sodium oxybate, GHB).

While the outcome of this therapeutic regime is considered adequate, in some patients it is not perfect. GHB, however, when used as a hypnotic is very effective when taken at bedtime.

GHB when used to treat narcolepsy was found to do the following.

1. Decrease the time to sleep.
2. Does not alter REM sleep.

If a drug does not alter REM sleep, there is no rebound or need for more REM sleep as is seen with some of the sedative hypnotics.

GHB was also tested as an adjuvant to anesthetics and the results were very positive, but its use never really caught on. It has been examined for possible therapeutic use for a number of other disorders, but due to the alleged ability to produce euphoria, hypnosis, and sedation, and since the number of illicit or dangerous episodes had increased, its use as a therapeutic agent decreased. GHB is still approved for use in the treatment of narcolepsy and has been given a Schedule III rating; however, it was also given a Schedule I rating and considered a drug of abuse (U.S. Federal Register, 2000).

CLINICAL USE OF γ HYDROXYBUTYRATE: TREATMENT OF ALCOHOL AND HEROIN ADDICTION

Preclinical and clinical studies began in Italy to determine if GHB blocked the more severe symptoms of withdrawal from alcohol, such as tremor, anxiety, and depression.

Studies in Animals

GHB was considered as a potential aid in the treatment of alcoholism. The rational for this treatment was based primarily on the findings in animal studies. In these studies, rats were made physically dependent on alcohol. When the alcohol-dependent rats were deprived of alcohol, it was observed that the withdrawal symptoms were less intense when the rats were given GHB as a substitute drug. These findings suggested that GHB could be used to suppress or reduce the intensity of the alcohol withdrawal symptoms. When GHB was administered acutely to rats, there was a 70% decrease in voluntary alcohol intake. It was also noted that a cross-tolerance to GHB developed, suggesting that there was a common neural substrate between GHB and alcohol, or even that GHB may mimic or potentiate the effects of alcohol.

Studies in Humans

There have been several large studies using GHB to suppress the symptoms of alcohol withdrawal. While all of the studies were not well controlled, several findings became clear. (1) GHB was effective in promoting abstinence. (2) GHB did decrease withdrawal symptoms. Many of the studies were performed over a period of 1 week so it is difficult to determine the final outcome with regard to promoting abstinence from alcohol. However, at the end of these studies, some of the patients had apparently developed an addiction to GHB, and were exhibiting symptoms of GHB withdrawal (Dyer et al., 2001; Addolorato et al., 2000).

GHB was also examined for its ability to suppress the withdrawal syndrome produced by heroin and methadone (Gallimberti et al., 1993). Patients were hospitalized and given GHB every 2–6 hours. There was a significant decrease in the withdrawal syndrome normally produced by these two drugs. At the end of 8 days, patients were given naloxone (an antagonist of heroin or methadone) and there was no observed response to naloxone (If patients were still using heroin, there would have been a very marked withdrawal syndrome develop.). The conclusion drawn from these studies was that GHB was potentially useful in alleviating many of the withdrawal symptoms produced by heroin.

Recent studies using GHB as a substitute drug are more highly controlled due to the abuse potential. Contrary to earlier studies, it is now recognized that GHB can produce both mental and physical addiction and that there is a high abuse liability associated with the use of GHB (for review, see McDonough et al., 2004; Carter et al., 2009). Even though it does suppress withdrawal symptoms for both alcohol and heroin, there is the potential of simply substituting another addicting drug. In a recent clinical study, a patient was administered baclofen for GHB withdrawal. Since the withdrawal symptoms were alleviated, the authors concluded that GABA$_B$ receptors mediated the dependence-producing symptoms (LeTourneau et al., 2008). These findings may prove very useful in developing a treatment for other addictions, such as alcoholism.

ABUSE POTENTIAL

There have been numerous clinical reports on the development of physical dependence following frequent use of GHB. Initial studies reported that neither tolerance nor dependence developed with the use of GHB; more recently, it has been demonstrated that dependence does develop and the withdrawal symptoms can be very severe (Andresen et al., 2011).

In the 1990s, GHB could be bought over the counter at health food stores and was used by body builders to increase muscle mass. GHB has a known releasing effect on growth hormone and was considered to be the "fountain of youth" drug. At roughly the same time, rumors started, suggesting that it also produced euphoria and GHB was being used in clubs as a "date rape" drug. When GHB was added to an alcoholic drink, the alcohol potentiated the effect of GHB. The result of this combination was a very rapid intoxication and usually the girl would pass out. When she woke, she rarely had any memory of what had happened. GHB soon became known as the "date rape" drug, and was now considered in the group of club drugs, along with methamphetamine, ketamine, and Rohypnol (Gahlinger, 2004). This use of GHB reached a peak in the late 1990s, at which time severe restrictions were put on the drug. The effects of GHB, even at low doses, when taken with alcohol, were potentially life threatening. People would go into a coma that could last for several hours. Because of the CNS depressant action, most people required being taken to the emergency room. In spite of these findings, GHB was still given an orphan drug approval for use in the treatment of narcolepsy.

As with benzodiazepines, the management of GHB overdose consists of supplying supportive measures for the following symptoms.

1. A decrease in respiration.
2. A decrease in heart rate.
3. A decrease in blood pressure.
4. CNS depression reversed by physostigmine or anticholinergics.

PHARMACOKINETICS

When taken orally, GHB reaches peak plasma levels in 1.5–2 hours. This long latency to peak effect will often cause a user to take a second dose thinking they have not taken enough GHB; this second dose may constitute an overdose. GHB has a duration of action of approximately 3 hours and the half-life varies in humans between 35 minutes and 2.7 hours.

GHB produces a dose-dependent response and this response is nonlinear. Even at very low doses GHB has been shown to produce death in humans, possibly due to co-administration with other drugs. GHB is metabolized by the P450 system.

> ## Review Questions
>
> 1. GHB affects many neurotransmitter systems. Describe the systems and the effect of GHB on those systems.
> 2. What over-the-counter use for GHB is no longer legal?
> 3. How is GHB overdose managed?

REFERENCES AND ADDITIONAL READING

Addolorato G, Caputo F, Capristo E, Stefanini GF, Gasbarrini G. 2000. Gamma hydroxybutyric acid: efficacy, potential abuse and dependence in the treatment of alcohol addiction. *Alcohol.* 20:217–222.

Andresen H, Aydin BE, Mueller A, Iwersen-Bergmann S. 2011. An overview of gamma-hydroxybutyric acid: pharmacodynamics, pharmacokinetics, toxic effect, addiction, analytical methods and interpretation of results. *Drug. Test. Anal.* 3:560–568.

Benavides J, Rumigny JF, Bourguignon JJ, et al. 1982. High affinity binding sites for g-hydroxybutyric acid in rat brain. *Life. Sci.* 30:953–961.

Carter LP, Koek W, France CP. 2009. Behavioral analyses of GHB: receptor mechanisms. *Pharmacol. Ther.* 12:100–114.

Crunelli V, Leresche N. 2002. Action of γ-hydroxybutyric on neuronal excitability and underlying membrane conductances. In: Tunnincliff G, Cash CD (eds), Gamma Hydroxybutyrate. Taylor & Francis Press, pp. 75–110.

Crunelli V, Emri Z, Leresche N. 2005. Unraveling the brain targets of gamma-hydroxybutyric acid. *Curr. Opin. Pharmacol.* 6:44–52.

Dahlstrom A, Fuxe K. 1964. Evidence for the existence of monoamine-containing neurons in the central nervous system. I. Demonstration of monoamines in the cell bodies of brain stem neurons. *Acta. Physiol. Scand.* 62(suppl. 232): 1–55.

Dyer JE, Roth B, Hyma BA. 2001. Gamma-hydroxybutyrate withdrawal syndrome. *Ann. Emerg. Med.* 37:147–153.

Fuller DE, Hornfeldt CS. 2003. From club drug to orphan drug: sodium oxybate (Xyrem) for the treatment of cataplexy. *Pharmacotherapy.* 23:1205–1209.

Gahlinger PM. 2004. Gamma-Hydroxybutyrate (GHB), Rohypnol, and Ketamine. *Am. Fam. Physician.* 69:2619–2626.

Gallimberti I, Cibin M, Pagnin P, et al. 1993. Gamma-hydroxybutyric acid for treatment of opiate withdrawal syndrome. *Neuropsychopharmacology.* 9:77–81.

Howard SG, Banerjee PK. 2002. Regulation of central dopamine by γ-hydroxybutyrate. In: Tunnicliff G, Cash CD (eds), *Gamma-Hydroxybutyrate: Molecular, Functional and Clinical Aspects.* Taylor & Francis, London and New York, pp. 111–119.

Laborit L. 1964. Sodium 4-hydroxybutyrate. *J. Neuropharmacol.* 32:433–451.

Laborit H, Jouany JM, Gerard J, Fabiani F. 1960. Summary of an experimental and clinical study on a metabolic substrate with inhibitory central action: sodium 4-hydroxybutyrate. *Presse. Med.* 68:1867–1869.

LeTourneau J, Hagg DS, Smith SM. 2008. Baclofen and gamma-hydroxybutyrate withdrawal. *Neurocrit. Care.* 8:430–433.

Maitre M. 1997. The gamma-hydroxybutyrate, signaling system in brain: organization and functional implications. *Prog. Neurobiol.* 51:337–361.

McDonough M, Kennedy N, Glasper A, Bearn J. 2004. Clinical features and management of gamma-hydroxybutyrate (GHV) withdrawal: a review. *Drug. Alcohol. Depend.* 75:3–9.

Snead OC. 1991. The gamma-hydroxybutyrate model of generalized absence seizures: correlation of regional brain levels of gamma-hydroxybutyric acid and gamma-butyrolactone with spike wave discharges. *Neuropharmacology.* 30:161–167.

Snead OC. 1994. The 3rd relation of the [3H] γ-hydroxybutyric acid (GHB) binding sites: relation to the development of experimental absence seizures. *Brain Res.* 52:1235–1243.

United States Federal Register. Schedules of controlled substances: addition of g-hydroxybutyric acid to Schedule I. Drug Enforcement Administration. Department of Justice. Final rule. *Fed Regist.* 2000:65:21645–21647.

Wu Y., Ali S, Ahmadian G, et al. 2004. γ-IIydroxybutyric acid (GHB) and g-aminobutyric acid receptor (GABAB$_R$) binding sites are distinctive from one another: molecular evidence. *Neuropharmacology.* 47:1146–1156.

Part IV Analgesics

Part IV Antigens

8 Morphine and Morphine Analogs

Carlos Cepeda

Learning Objectives

The student will learn:

1. Historical aspects of the use of opioids over the centuries.
2. The mechanism of action of morphine, the prototype opioid.
3. The action of the opioid receptors and their distribution in the body.
4. The central and peripheral effects of morphine and heroin.
5. Why heroin is so addictive.
6. The role of glutamate receptors in the formation of a physical dependence to opioids.
7. The central and peripheral effects of the antagonists, naloxone and naltrexone.

Humans are genetically programmed to avoid pain. However, for better or for worse, pain is our perennial companion from the moment of birth until death. While the sensation of pain undoubtedly has an adaptive value as a harbinger of impending danger or disease, most people would do anything to escape its powerful grip. The euphoria caused by pain relief appears to be more intense than sexual pleasure and more addictive than cocaine. Throughout human history, the search for better and stronger painkillers began early and continues unabated. Even our own brain possesses endogenous chemicals, called endorphins, with the ability to diminish pain.

Ingestion of painkillers can be extremely addictive. The problem of addiction to opiates has increased to such a degree that in a recent study an increase was found in the number of babies being born with opiate withdrawal syndrome, due to exposure *in utero* to painkillers. In Canada,

Drugs of Abuse: Pharmacology and Molecular Mechanisms, First Edition. Sherrel G. Howard.
© 2014 John Wiley & Sons, Inc. Published 2014 by John Wiley & Sons, Inc.

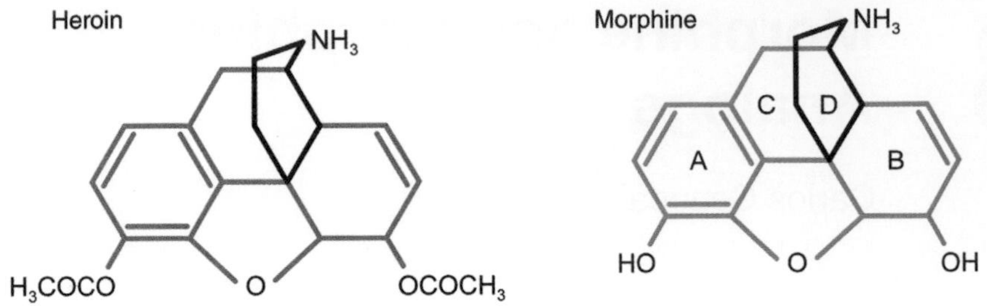

Heroin

Morphine

Figure 8.1   Structural formula for morphine and heroin.

when OxyContin was banned, pharmacies were burglarized at gunpoint in search of the last doses of the painkiller.

Morphine, heroin, and the strongest prescription drugs to treat pain, are derived from opium (Figure 8.1). The term opioid applies to any substance, whether endogenous or synthetic, that produces a morphine-like effect, which can be blocked by antagonists such as naloxone.

HISTORY OF OPIOIDS

Opium (*Papaver somniferum*) is an extract of the poppy seed that has been used for thousands of years. The earliest record of its use was in Sumeria, dating back to the fourth millennium BC. The Sumerians called opium "the joy plant." Written records were found in Assyria dating back to the seventh century BC describing the method of collecting opium, which is basically the same method that is used today. The art of opium cultivation was then passed on to the Babylonians and the Egyptians, who initiated production of opium as well as the profitable trade of the plant around the world.

Opium is referred to in "The Iliad," where Helen mixed a potion of "freedom from grief and pain." Everyone from Hippocrates to Galen described its various medicinal uses. While the Father of Medicine dismissed the magical attributes of opium, he acknowledged it was a powerful narcotic, and Avicenna of Persia described it as the most powerful stupefacient. Indian medical treatises recommended the use of opium for diarrhea and sexual debility. Paracelsus introduced laudanum, also known as "stones of immortality," as a powerful painkiller.

By the seventeenth century opium was a common ingredient in many potions throughout Europe. Fortunately, there were so many ingredients in these potions that very little harm was caused to the patient. Thomas Sydenham, an English apothecary, mixed opium with sherry wine and herbs, and called his concoction "Sydenham's laudanum," which rapidly became a popular remedy for numerous ailments. Unfortunately, along with its widespread use in medicine, came a surge of opium consumption for recreational purposes. The medical profession was worried about the lavish use of opium during the 1700s, but their warnings were largely ignored.

During the early 1800s, the German pharmacist Friedrich Wilhelm Sertürner isolated a pure alkaloid base from opium. In 1805, in a letter to the editor of a local journal, he reported the isolation from opium of a substance that showed alkaline properties. However, he was largely ignored. Undaunted, Sertürner continued research work on this substance and in 1817 he published again his results introducing additional observations made in humans and for the first time called it "Morphine" for the God of sleep. This time his publication was greatly acknowledged. The famous chemist Louis Gay-Lussac ordered a translation into French, which finally earned Sertürner widespread recognition. In 1832, Pierre Jean Bobiquet isolated codeine (3-methylmorphine), the second most prevalent alkaloid in opium. In 1835, another French chemist, Pierre Pelletier, isolated thebaine.

In 1657, the renowned architect Christopher Wren invented what, after some refinements, would become the hypodermic needle. It was thought that intravenous (IV) injections would make introduction of substances easier if they could be put directly into a vein. Documents show that he first experimented with dogs injecting them with opium. However, the needle that was used had a blunt end so that injections had to be preceded by cutting through the skin with a knife and then the needle was inserted into the vein. Some years later the beveled edge was introduced. The French physician Charles Pravaz designed the hypodermic needle in 1853. The syringe was made out of silver and operated by a screw, rather than a plunger, to control the amount of substance injected. That same year, Alexander Wood, a physician from Edinburgh, invented the first hypodermic needle that used a true syringe and a hollow needle, taking the sting of the bee as his model. He was able to administer morphine, finding the effects to be instantaneous and three times more potent. Hypodermic needles were initially used for injecting morphine as a painkiller, as physicians erroneously believed that this drug would not be addictive if it bypassed the digestive tract. Ironically, rumor says that Woods's wife became the first morphine needle addict.

During the American Civil War, there was such widespread use of morphine and the hypodermic syringe that addiction to morphine was called the "Soldiers Disease." It is believed that as many as 4000 soldiers were addicted. In fact, morphine use in the nineteenth century was so widespread that it was given to infants and children in the form of "Mrs. Winslow's Soothing Syrup." It was advertised as a cure for painful teething, inflammation, regulation of the bowels, and of course, for colds and coughs. The advertisements picture idealized scenes of mother and child that were aimed at the "perfect" mother. However, children actually died due to the excessive use of Mrs. Winslow's Syrup by overprotective mothers. The Pure Food and Drug Act, a precursor of the FDA, was passed in 1906 due in part to Mrs. Winslow's Syrup (Figure 8.2).

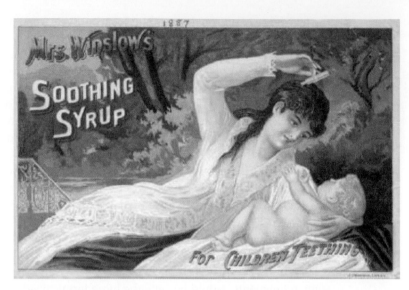

Figure 8.2   Winslow's Soothing Syrup. Private collection of S. Howard.

Control of opium production and trade has been a long-standing issue among different countries and cultures. In the 17th Century from 1637 onwards opium represented the main commodity of British trade with China. In 1729, Chinese emperor Yung Cheng issued an edict prohibiting domestic sales or smoking of opium. For several centuries the British controlled the opium trade from India and Turkey to China, Europe, and the United States. Smuggling made the fortunes of many people in America in the late nineteenth and early twentieth centuries. During World War II, countries of southeast Asia, the "Golden Triangle" formed by Laos, Thailand, and Burma, became major producers in the profitable opium trade. Now Afghanistan, Colombia, and Mexico are the main opium producers.

Attempts to curb opium consumption for recreational purposes are as old as civilization. Prescription drugs using opioids are the most abused drugs after tobacco and alcohol. The drug consumption in the United States and Canada is greater than all other countries combined. In the United States, between 1994 and 2002, the number of emergency room visits related to heroin consumption almost doubled, while that related to opiate therapeutics almost tripled. Taken together, the use of opiates in one form or another does not appear to be an easily solvable problem in society. However, an understanding of the effects of addiction on people's health and well-being may help to dissuade future users of opiates.

MECHANISM OF ACTION

Opioids act as agonists at the three opioid receptors. The binding sites are distributed widely throughout the central nervous system (CNS). The

Table 8.1 Opioid Drugs Interact at the Various Receptor Subtypes

β-endorphin	$+3\,\mu$, $+3\,\delta$, $+1\,\kappa$		
Enkephalin	$+2\,\mu$, $+3\,\delta$, $-\kappa$		
Dynorphin	$+2\,\mu$, $+2\,\delta$, $+3\,\kappa$		
Endomorphin	$+3\,\mu$, $-\delta$, $-\kappa$		
Pure Agonists	μ	δ	κ
Morphine	$+3$	$+1$	$+1$
DAMGO	$+3$	$+1$	$-$
DPDPE	$-$	$+3$	$-$
Enadoline	$-$	$-$	$+3$
Partial/Mixed Agonists			
Methadone	$+3$	$+2$	$+2$
Nalorphine	$+2$	$+2$	$+2$
Buprenorphine	$+3$	$+2$	$+2$
Antagonists			
Naloxone	$+3$		$+2$
Naltrexone	$+3$		$+3$
CTAP	$\dashv 3$		
Naltrindole		$+3$	
Nor-binaltorphimine			$+3$

$+1$ equals the smallest effect; $+3$ equals the biggest effect.

greatest numbers of binding sites occur in the limbic system (frontal and temporal cortex, amygdala, and hippocampus). There are also large numbers of binding sites in the spinal cord, thalamus, striatum, and hypothalamus. For the most part, the affinity of the particular opioid for the receptor reflects the potency of the analgesic action (Table 8.1).

OPIOID RECEPTORS

All opioid receptors are G-protein coupled receptors (GPCRs). There are three principal types of opioid receptors named after the first Greek letter of the preferred ligand or the site where it was characterized as μ (for morphine), δ (found in the vas deferens), and κ (for ketocyclazocine) (Figure 8.3). The existence of an orphan receptor (opioid-like receptor, OLR-1) has been proposed, based on cDNA homology. μ receptors are responsible for analgesia and also for some of the unwanted effects of morphine. δ receptors are more important in the periphery, while κ receptors induce analgesia at the level of the spinal cord and sedation. It has been suggested that each type of receptor has different subtypes such as μ ($\mu1$ and $\mu2$), δ ($\delta1$, $\delta2$ and $\delta3$), κ ($\kappa1$, $\kappa2$ and $\kappa3$). However, the evidence is still controversial, and other mechanisms such as alternative splicing and formation of receptor dimers have to be taken into account. To date, only one type of ORL-1 receptor has been found.

The distribution of μ-opioid receptors displays close overlap with the regions that enable pain perception (Table 8.2).

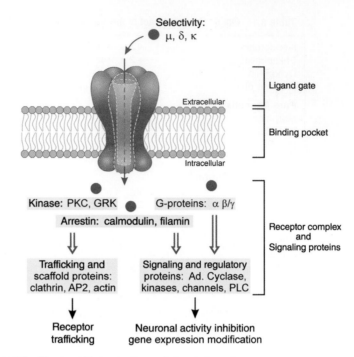

Figure 8.3   The morphine receptor and signal cascade.

Except for ORL-1 receptors, all other receptor types produce some de-gree of analgesia (Table 8.3). There is a general consensus that μ-opioid re-ceptors mediate the classical beneficial and adverse effects of opiate drugs. For example, mice lacking μ-opioid receptors display no morphine anal-gesia or conditioned place preference (CPP, a behavioral test widely used to explore the reinforcing effects of drugs that produce addiction. It oc-curs when a subject learns to prefer one place more than others because the site has been associated with rewarding events). The powerful sense of well-being and the sudden rush induced by morphine or heroin given

Table 8.2   The Distribution of μ-Opioid Receptors Displays Close Overlap with the Regions That Enable Pain Perception

μ Receptors found in:	δ Receptors found in:	κ Receptors found in:
Substantia gelatinosa	Pontine nuclei	Hypothalamus
Periaqueductal gray	Olfactory bulb	Periaqueductal gray
Reticular formation	Cerebral cortex	Claustrum
Hypothalamus	Peripheral sensory neurons	Substantia gelatinosa
Thalamus		Peripheral sensory neurons
Cerebral cortex		

The ORL-1 receptors are found in cortex, amygdala, hippocampus, septal nuclei, habenula, hypothalamus, and spinal cord.

Table 8.3 Functional Effects Associated with Opioid Receptors

	μ	δ	κ
Analgesia	+3	+2	–
Respiratory depression	+3	+1	–
Pupil constriction	+3	–	+1
Euphoria	+3	–	–
Dysphoria			+3
Physical dependence	+3		

+1 equals the smallest effect; +3 equals the greatest effect.

IV are mainly mediated through the μ receptor. Analgesia and respiratory depression are also mediated by these receptors. Respiratory depression is the most unwanted and troublesome side effect of the analgesic drugs, outside of addiction, and it occurs at therapeutic doses.

Animal studies showed that δ agonists, although analgesic, may also induce epileptic seizures and κ agonists could be dysphoric and possibly hallucinogenic. However, receptor distribution varies among species and it is unclear if those effects also occur in humans. The ORL-1 is not considered a classical opioid receptor. However, some opiate drugs used in the clinic do bind to these receptors.

In 1992, two groups, one led by Chris Evans at UCLA and the other by Brigitte Kieffers in Strassbourg, independently cloned the δ-opioid receptor. Soon thereafter, other groups cloned the μ and κ receptors. While the atomic structure of opioid receptors had eluded crystallography, in 2012 the structure of μ and κ receptors was finally elucidated. Ray Stevens' lab at Scripps Research Institute in La Jolla, and Kobilka and Granier's lab at Stanford, demonstrated that the binding pockets of both receptors are large and gaping which, according to Stevens, could explain how the κ-opioid receptor recognizes a diverse set of molecules. Kobilka and Granier say that the openness of the μ-receptor-binding site could explain why the actions of opioids can turn on so quickly and be rapidly reversed by appropriate antagonists.

CENTRAL NERVOUS SYSTEM EFFECTS

Morphine has both stimulant and depressant effects on the CNS and there is a great variation in the degree to which this occurs. The effects of morphine and other opioids are very diverse and range from analgesia, drowsiness, changes in mood to respiratory depression, decreased gastrointestinal (GI) motility and changes in the autonomic system. For example, cats become extremely excited by morphine, while the effect in humans is generally one of sedation. This is not always the case, however, as some humans do become excited by morphine.

Morphine also produces dizziness, a sensation of warmth, itching, and nausea. Nausea and vomiting occur in up to 40% of patients who receive morphine. The nausea is due primarily to stimulation of chemoreceptors in the trigger zone of the medulla oblongata, which activates emetic centers, and the orthostatic hypotension that is also produced by morphine. Other secondary effects of morphine include a big reduction of the affective components associated with pain. Thus, even if you feel pain, it does not bother you. This probably reflects an action at the level of the limbic system. When injected IV morphine produces a powerful feeling of euphoria. There are also undesirable and sometimes lethal side effects including respiratory depression, constipation (which occurs at therapeutic doses), reduction in the cough reflex and bronco-constriction, which puts asthmatics at grave risk.

The main sympathetic nervous system effects include bradycardia, orthostatic hypotension, and reduction of the immune response in long-term users (see Table 8.3 for a comparison of the functional effects obtained from stimulation of different opioid receptors). Morphine does increase cerebrospinal fluid (CSF) pressure also leading to respiratory depression. In addition, morphine produces myosis (constriction of the pupils) in species where the drug is a sedative and mydriasis (dilated pupils) if it produces excitation. Morphine also increases tone and decreases motility in many parts of the GI system.

Morphine is effective for both acute and chronic pain. Interestingly it is not a good local anesthetic and is generally ineffective for use in neuropathic pain syndromes (i.e., phantom limb and/or trigeminal neuralgia).

ENDOGENOUS MORPHINE

Hans Kosterlitz, from Scotland, in collaboration with his younger colleague John Hughes, is credited with the discovery of endogenous substances in the brain (enkephalins) that produce effects similar to those of morphine. Ironically, the experiment that led to this discovery was envisioned in one of his dreams while in the arms of Morpheus. He stimulated a strip of guinea pig intestine electrically and recorded the contractions with a polygraph. He then found that if opiates were added to the solution, intestinal contractions would stop. More importantly, application of a pig brain cell homogenate produced the same effect. Interestingly, recent studies have demonstrated that animal and human tissues are capable of producing morphine itself.

The family of endogenous ligands for the opioid receptors is called endorphins. They are produced by the pituitary gland and the hypothalamus. The main triggers of endorphin release are pain and stress. Other stimuli include exercise, consumption of spicy food, sex, and orgasm. Endorphins do not produce euphoria directly, even though we hear about runner's high. Alcohol consumption also induces endogenous opioid release in nucleus accumbens and orbitofrontal cortex. Further, changes in the cortex correlate with alcohol use and subjective high in heavy drinkers. This suggests a possible mechanism by which opioid antagonists can be used to treat alcohol abuse.

Endorphins are produced by three large precursor molecules:

1. Proenkephalin
2. Prodynorphin
3. Proopiomelanocortin

These three molecules generate a multitude of endogenous opioid neuropeptides. Proopiomelanocortin transcripts are found in the pituitary, the arcuate nucleus, and cells of the solitary tract. Proenkephalin and prodynorphin are more widely distributed throughout the brain.

To reduce the level of perceived pain, endogenous opioids (enkephalins, dynorphin) are released by interneurons in the dorsal horn in response to severe pain. The opioids bind to G proteins associated with μ-opioid receptors, which leads to inhibition of pre-synaptic release of glutamate and increased K^+ conductance at the post-synaptic membrane. The enkephalins preferentially bind δ receptors, while endorphins and endomorphins bind μ receptors and dynorphin binds κ receptors. Nociceptin is the endogenous ligand for the ORL-1 receptor.

Opioids have probably been studied more intensively than any other group of drugs in an effort to understand their powerful effects in molecular, biochemical, and physiological terms, as well as in an attempt to develop opioid drugs with analgesic properties but with advantages over morphine. While we understand its interaction at various receptor subtypes, we still do not know the intimate physiological pathways that are regulated by morphine, and which underlie the analgesic effects of morphine. However, in the last few years, significant advances in the knowledge of receptor structure and intracellular cascades have occurred, giving us a better idea of the mechanisms involved in opioids' effects.

The classic view of opioid receptors as on/off switches is changing in favor of a complex and dynamic sensing system capable of orchestrating the interaction of different proteins (Walwyn et al., 2010). Receptor trafficking is regulated by endogenous and synthetic ligands. While many opioid agonists induce μ-opioid receptor internalization, morphine itself does not. However, increasing levels of β-arrestins (binding receptor proteins that, after agonist activation, arrest or stop further signaling) can enhance internalization of μ receptors by morphine.

As previously mentioned, opioid receptors belong to the super-family of GPCRs. Opioid receptors

1. inhibit adenylate cyclase;
2. decrease cAMP content intracellularly;
3. promote opening of K^+ channels;
4. inhibit opening of voltage-gated Ca^{2+} channels.

These actions reduce membrane excitability of neurons as well as neurotransmitter release. So the overall effect at the cellular level is inhibitory. Interestingly, chronic opiate use leads to an increase in Ca^{2+} influx through N-methyl-D-aspartate (NMDA) receptors as well as increased expression of Ca^{2+}/calmodulin-dependent protein kinase II (CaMKII), cCMP response element-binding protein (CREB) phosphorylation, and c-fos messenger RNA (mRNA) expression, which could be responsible for neuroadaptations manifested as synaptic plasticity (Noda and Nabeshima, 2004). Morphine also releases histamine from mast cells. This is unrelated to the receptors, but is responsible for the urticaria or itching that often occurs with these drugs.

While the analgesic effect of μ-opioid receptor agonists is due to direct inhibitory effects on pain transmission at the spinal cord and descending pain-modulating pathways, the rewarding effects are partially due to dopamine release by ventral tegmental area (VTA) neurons innervating the nucleus accumbens. Although the reinforcing effects of opiates involve both dopamine-dependent and dopamine-independent mechanisms, there is no doubt that the reward system plays a critical role in opiate dependence. Recent studies have demonstrated differential actions of direct (dopamine D_1 receptor-expressing) and indirect (dopamine D_2 receptor-expressing) medium-sized spiny neurons (MSNs) in the nucleus accumbens. Thus, the μ agonist DAMGO reduced excitatory synaptic input onto D_2 cells, whereas it concurrently decreased inhibitory input onto D_1 MSNs (Ma et al., 2012). This suggests different roles of direct and indirect pathway MSNs in opiate effects. Furthermore, ablation of D_2 cells led to increased amphetamine CPP, indicating that indirect pathway MSNs limit drug reinforcement (Durieux et al., 2009). By extension, it is possible that direct pathway cells facilitate drug reinforcement and addiction, thus recapitulating the general plan of motor behavior regulation by the neostriatum (Ma et al., 2012).

The effects of morphine on central neurons are diverse and depend on multiple factors such as the neuronal subtype and the cerebral region under investigation. Although most studies found depressing effects, other studies have reported excitatory effects from morphine. In general, opioids reduce neurotransmitter release by presynaptic mechanisms. However, postsynaptically, they may increase neuronal excitability. For example, morphine changes the regular firing pattern of cortical pyramidal neurons into a bursting mode, which could explain epileptic activity induced by high doses of morphine.

In addition, the effects of morphine can be at odds with those of endogenous ligands. This led to the suggestion that opioid compounds act not as neurotransmitters but as neuromodulators of synaptic activity and excitability. It is also known that chronic administration of opiates induces structural changes in neurons, including changes in the number of dendritic spines in cortex and hippocampus.

HEROIN

In 1874, C. R. Wright, an English researcher, boiling morphine over a stove, synthesized heroin (diacetylmorphine) (Figure 8.1). As the chemical name suggests, heroin is formed by adding two acetyl groups to morphine. Heroin was named after the German word for powerful or heroic. Commercial production began in 1898 and was initially advertised by Bayer as "the sedative for coughs." This "miracle" drug was a bestseller for several years and doctors were unaware of the potential addictive properties of heroin. However, they soon realized that some of their patients were consuming excessive amounts of cough remedies and in 1913 the company halted heroin production.

What most people experience after heroin consumption is

1. a sense of protection;
2. a warm feeling of relaxation;
3. dissipation of pain;
4. reduced fear, hunger, and anxiety.

Heroin is particularly addictive because it enters the brain so quickly due to acetyl groups, which confer increased lipid solubility and allow crossing the blood–brain barrier more quickly. Heroin, if injected, reaches the brain within 15 seconds and, if smoked, in just 7 seconds. With heroin the rush is usually accompanied by a warm flushing of the skin, dry mouth, and a heavy feeling in the extremities, which may be accompanied by nausea, vomiting, and severe itching. Addicts feel tired initially and mental function is clouded for several hours. Cardiac function slows down as does breathing, sometimes to the point of death. In fact, in many cases heroin overdose involves suppression of respiration. Its continuous use during pregnancy can lead to reduced childbirth weight and developmental delays. In some cases it can also cause spontaneous abortion.

Because the vast majority of addicts use needles to self-administer heroin, this is associated with additional risks such as infectious diseases, HIV/AIDS, hepatitis B and C, collapsed veins, abscesses, and infections of the heart, valves, and lining of the heart.

PRESCRIPTION DRUGS

The bases for most painkillers and cough suppressants are alkaloids found in opium. Prominent among them are morphine itself, codeine, and thebaine. Codeine is the most widely used opiate in the world, mainly for medicinal but also recreational purposes.

Codeine

Codeine is used chiefly to relieve cough and to treat moderate pain. It can be used in isolation or combined with other analgesics. Common side effects of codeine include euphoria, itching, nausea, dry mouth, and constipation. As with other opioid drugs, respiratory depression occurs and it can have fatal consequences. Tolerance and physical dependence also develop after chronic use of codeine compounds. Cough suppression does not correlate with analgesia, such that sub-analgesic doses of codeine can effectively suppress cough. This is why codeine was used in cough syrup for so long and was then replaced with dextromethorphan.

Thebaine

Thebaine (paramorphine) is similar to morphine and codeine but it has stimulatory rather than depressant effects. At high doses it can produce convulsions. However, an enantiomer of thebaine does have analgesic effects. Although as such it is not used in the clinic, thebaine can be industrially converted into a wide range of opioid agonists including oxycodone, orymorphone, buprenorphine, etorphine, and antagonists such as naloxone and naltrexone.

Oxycodone

Oxycodone was developed by Freund and Speyer in Germany in 1916 and is generally prescribed for pain relief. It was introduced in the US market in 1939. In 1998, oxycodone production worldwide was about 11.5 tons, by 2007 this figure jumped to 75.2 tons. The United States has the highest per capita consumption of oxycodone, about 82% of the world total. While it is no substitute for morphine in cases of severe pain, it produces less respiratory depression and other undesirable side effects. However, it is not innocuous as it can produce memory loss, fatigue, dizziness, nausea, itching, and sweating. Sudden removal of the drug, as would be expected, can lead to withdrawal symptoms.

OxyContin

OxyContin, manufactured by Purdue Pharma, is the brand name of a time-release formula of oxycodone. It is estimated that OxyContin is the best-selling narcotic pain reliever, with about $2.5 billion in sales in the United States alone. Purdue Pharma has been accused of misleading the public about the potential risks of the drug. In fact, the company had to pay millions in fines for aggressive marketing practices and misrepresentation. The abuse risks were so prominent that in 2011 the company included an abuse-resistant polymer that decreased its recreational use. Roxane Laboratories produce a new formulation of oxycodone that has become the new choice of drug abusers. They are known by their street names as Roxies, Blues, Berries, and "30's" (for the 30 mg dose).

PHARMACOKINETICS

The plasma half-life of morphine is 3–6 hours. Morphine is metabolized by glucuronidase producing morphine-6-glucuronide. This metabolite of morphine has more analgesic properties than morphine. Heroin has similar half-life as morphine.

Codeine converts into morphine in the liver, a reaction that is catalyzed by the cytochrome P450 enzyme CYP2D6. CYP3A4 produces norcodeine and UGT2B7 conjugates codeine, norcodeine, and morphine to the corresponding 3- and 6-glucuronides. Oxycodone has a higher oral bioavailability and is about twice as potent as morphine. It does not require conversion to oxymorphone for pharmacological activity.

Opiate Tolerance

Both physical and psychological tolerance to opiates develops 12–24 hours after acute injection. Tolerance can be demonstrated by the hot plate technique, and measuring how long it takes mice to jump off of the hot plate. Standard hot plate tests take 3 days to return to normal. Tolerance can be developed to analgesia, emesis, euphoria, and respiratory depression. An addicted person can take 50 times the initial therapeutic dose without experiencing respiratory depression. Cross-tolerance occurs between drugs (opioids) acting at the same receptor, but not between opioids acting at different receptors.

PHYSICAL DEPENDENCE AND WITHDRAWAL SYNDROME

Physical dependence is characterized by a craving for the drug and rather pronounced symptoms if the drug is withdrawn. The Abstinence syndrome that occurs on abrupt withdrawal of the drug is similar across species. In mice, withdrawal leads to increased irritability, loss of weight, body shakes, tremors, writhing, jumping, and aggression. Abrupt withdrawal in humans induces several signs reminiscent of severe influenza including yawning, fever, sweating, piloerection, nausea, diarrhea, and insomnia.

Glutamate NMDA receptors play a critical role in opioid physical dependence. Indeed, there is a positive association between expression of NMDA receptor subunits and addictive behavior. Using the CPP model, a robust increase in NR2B subunits was demonstrated in the nucleus accumbens of rats conditioned by morphine (Ma et al., 2011). In agreement, Ifenprodil (a selective antagonist of NR2B-containing NMDA receptors) produced a dose-dependent reduction in reward craving induced by morphine (Ma et al., 2006). NR1 subunits are also involved in the development of morphine dependence (Noda and Nabeshima, 2004) and mice with knock out of NR2A subunits display reduced morphine withdrawal syndrome.

ANTAGONISTS OF MORPHINE

Naloxone was the first pure opioid antagonist with an affinity for all three of the principal opioid receptors. (For a comparison of activity at a given receptor, see Table 8.1.) It blocks the actions of endogenous opioid peptides, as well as those of morphine-like drugs and is also used as a tool to determine the physiological role of these peptides, particularly in pain transmission. Naloxone produces a rapid reversal of the effects of morphine and morphine-like compounds. It has little or no effect when given on its own to normal subjects. Also, it has little effect on the pain threshold under normal circumstances. However, under stress conditions or if there is inflammation when endogenous opioids are produced, for example, at the dentist's office, it produces hypoanalgesia. It is interesting to note that naloxone will also inhibit acupuncture-induced analgesia. The primary clinical use of naloxone is to treat respiratory depression caused by an overdose of any of the opioids. It is also occasionally used in newborns to reverse the effects of analgesics used during delivery to improve breathing. Then it is usually given IV and the effects occur immediately. The effect of naloxone lasts for ~2 to 4 hours, which is shorter than most morphine-like drugs, so it may have to be administered several times. Naloxone will precipitate withdrawal symptoms in addicts.

Naltrexone is structurally very similar to naloxone (Figure 8.4), but with a much longer duration of action. Its half-life is about 10 hours.

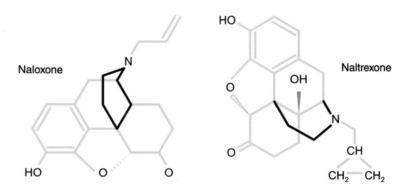

Figure 8.4   Structural formula for naloxone and naltrexone.

Naltrexone has been approved by the FDA as a maintenance drug. It will block virtually all effects of heroin. It is often said that it is of value to addicts who have been detoxified since it will nullify the effect of a dose of opiate should their resolve fail.

TREATMENT

Acute opioid intoxication or overdose can be treated with naloxone. As there is generally respiratory depression after opioid overdose, cardiac and pulmonary functions have to be monitored constantly. If needed, support ventilation has to be provided.

Pharmacologic attempts to treat drug addiction induced by opiates have achieved mild success but are still in use until better treatments become available. The main goal of this type of therapy is the amelioration of withdrawal symptoms and reduction of drug cravings. By replacing opiates with legally obtained agonists, risk factors associated with drug abuse can be partially mitigated. Methadone has been the gold standard for many years but the recent advent of buprenorphine maintenance therapy is changing the landscape of treatment for opioid-dependent patients. Methadone, a long-acting synthetic opioid agonist, can be taken once daily, however, it is a highly regulated Schedule II medication and is only available at specialized methadone maintenance clinics. Buprenorphine is a μ-opioid partial agonist that also suppresses withdrawal and cravings. What makes this drug superior to methadone is that partial agonist confers a "ceiling effect," meaning that higher doses cause no additional effects, thus affording a wider margin of safety than methadone, which can be lethal in overdose. Buprenorphine can be combined with naloxone in a 4:1 ratio (Suboxone). Extended-release intramuscular (IM) naltrexone (Depotrex) has been used for the prevention of relapse to opioid dependence with increased retention of patients under treatment.

Safe withdrawal from opioids is known as detoxification. A formulation combining methadone, buprenorphine, and α-2 agonists, such as clonidine and lofexidine, are commonly used for detoxification. The use of methadone and buprenorphine is based on the principle of cross-tolerance in which one opioid is replaced by another and then slowly withdrawn. α-2 agonists are effective in suppressing autonomic signs of abstinence.

Opiate dependence and the withdrawal syndrome can be treated with NMDA receptor antagonists: Co-administration of morphine and dizocilpine, via inhibition of CaMKII in the cingulate cortex, decreases the development of morphine dependence (Noda and Nabeshima, 2004). Similarly, memantine (an NMDA receptor antagonist with preference for extrasynaptic receptors) reduces opiate physical dependence in humans.

In addition to these pharmacological methods, immunotherapy as a way to prevent relapse has been attempted. Although the idea of an anti-opiate vaccine is not new, recent findings are gaining momentum and wider recognition. The basis for this vaccine is the production of antibodies that bind addictive drugs and their metabolites in the bloodstream and prevent them from entering the brain, where they produce their euphoric effects. For example, Mexican scientists Anton and Lef (2006) demonstrated that a morphine–tetanus toxoid vaccine was able to produce antibodies that reduced the acquisition of heroin self-administration in rats and Janda et al. (2011), at the Scripps Research Institute in La Jolla, showed that polyclonal antibodies produced by a vaccine with a heroin-like hapten linked to keyhole limpet hemocyanin (KLH), a carrier protein, had micromolar affinities to heroin and morphine but were nonetheless able to prevent the acquisition of heroin self-administration and the antinociceptive effects of heroin in rodents.

Obviously, successful therapies for opiate addiction cannot succeed unless important cognitive and behavioral changes occur. Cognitive behavior-based models are widely used in drug rehabilitation programs. These techniques allow patients to acquire specific skills for resisting substance use and teach coping skills to reduce problems related to drug use. Group therapy and support groups such as Narcotics Anonymous, seems to be particularly effective. Finally, aversion therapy involving pairing of aversive stimuli to cognitive images of opioid use has met some success.

Is it possible to separate pain relief from its rewarding effects? While the dream of finding selective drugs that produce analgesia without being addictive could someday become a reality, many scientists remain skeptical. But even if feasible, when the physical and psychological pains that inevitably accumulate throughout our lives become a heavy burden, do we really want to deprive human beings from the guilty pleasures associated with pain relief? At least in some cases, it should be justified to give pain-ridden people a few moments of relief and happiness with what Sir William Osler called "God's own medicine."

Review Questions

1. Discuss the role of the different opioid receptors.
2. What is the role of the glutamate receptors in opioid dependence?
3. What is the effect of naloxone on a non-addicted person?
4. Discuss the role of endorphins in the body (i.e., what are they, where are the receptors located, and what do they do).
5. Discuss opiate tolerance.

REFERENCES AND ADDITIONAL READING

Anton B, Leff P. 2006. A novel bivalent morphine/heroin vaccine that prevents relapse to heroin addiction in rodents. *Vaccine*. 24:3232–3240.

Booth M. 1996. *Opium: A History*. Simon & Schuster, Ltd.

Durieux PF, Bearzatto B, Guiducci S, et al. 2009. D2R striatopallidal neurons inhibit both locomotor and drug reward processes. *Nat. Neurosci.* 12:393–395.

Evans CJ. 2004. Secrets of the opium poppy revealed. *Neuropharmacology.* 47:293–299.

Janda KD, Treweek JB. 2011. Vaccines targeting drugs of abuse: is the glass half-empty or half-full? *Nat. Rev. Immunol.* 12:67–72.

Ma YY, Cepeda C, Cui CL. 2011. The role of striatal NMDA receptors in drug addiction. *Int. Rev. Neurobiol.* 89:131–146.

Ma YY, Cepeda C, Chatta P, Franklin L, Evans CJ, Levine MS. 2012. Regional and cell-type-specific effects of DAMGO on striatal D1 and D2 dopamine receptor-expressing medium-sized spiny neurons. *ASN Neuro.* 4(2):e00077.

Ma YY, Guo CY, Yu P, Lee DY, Han JS, Cui CL. 2006. The role of NR2B containing NMDA receptor in place preference conditioned with morphine and natural reinforcers in rats. *Exp. Neurol.* 200:343–355.

Noda Y, Nabeshima T. 2004. Opiate physical dependence and N-methyl-D-aspartate receptors. *Eur. J. Pharm.* 500:121–128.

Shen XY, Orson FM, Kosten TR. 2012. Vaccines against drug abuse. *Nature.* 91:60–70.

Waldhoer M, Bartlett SE, Whistler JL. 2004. Opioid receptors. *Ann. Rev. Biochem.* 73:953–990.

Walwyn W, Miotto KA, Evans CJ. 2010. Opioid pharmaceuticals and addiction: the issues, and research directions seeking solutions. *Drug Alcohol Depend.* 108:156–165.

Part V Hallucinogens

9 Lysergic Acid Diethylamide and Mescaline

Learning Objectives

The student will learn:

1. The required components of the mechanism of action of lysergic acid diethylamide (LSD).
2. The central nervous system effects of LSD, including the effects on different serotonin (5-HT) receptors.
3. The peripheral nervous system effects of LSD.
4. The different classes of hallucinogens.
5. Long-term effects of LSD, including hallucination persisting perception disorder (HPPD) or flashbacks.
6. What is "candy flipping" and what are the effects of this drug combination?
7. The mechanism of action of mescaline.
8. The central and peripheral nervous system effects of mescaline.

Lysergic acid diethylamide (LSD) is a member of a class of pharmacological agents that produce marked distortions and alterations in one's perception in the visual, auditory, and tactile senses. Many of these compounds are plant based, such as the ergot alkaloids, the peyote cactus which contains mescaline and the *teonanacatl* mushroom, which contains psilocybin.

Historically, hallucinogenic plants were used largely for social and religious rituals and their availability was limited by climate and soil conditions (Schultz and Hoffman, 1980). Epidemics of ergot poisoning often occurred during the Middle Ages and in fact still occur occasionally today (Lee, 2010). Ergot poisoning does not just produce a daffy horse in the middle of a field, it occurs most commonly in contaminated grain that is used for cereal. The symptoms not only include mental disturbances,

Drugs of Abuse: Pharmacology and Molecular Mechanisms, First Edition. Sherrel G. Howard.

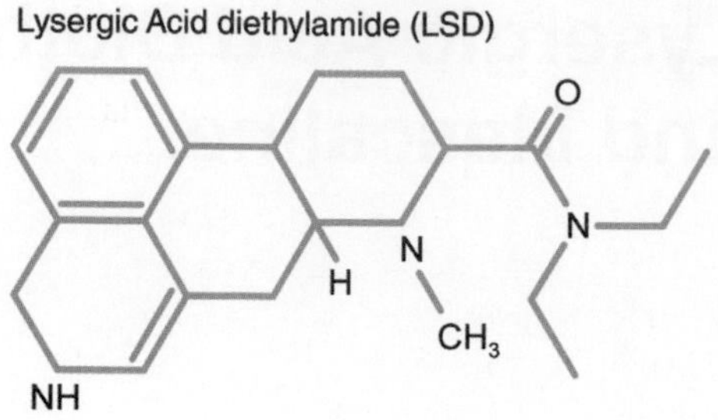

Lysergic Acid diethylamide (LSD)

Figure 9.1   Structure of lysergic acid diethylamide.

but also a very painful vasoconstriction that can lead to gangrene and potential loss of limbs. In the Middle Ages it was called, St. Anthony's fire, because it was usually cured by a visit to St. Anthony's shrine. Coincidentally, St. Anthony's shrine is located in a region of France that is ergot free (Medicinenet.com).

Ergot is a fungus that grows on wheat, barley, or rye, and is poisonous. However, midwives in Europe used ergot to induce labor. Ergotamine was isolated and purified in the early 1900s. It was widely used to stop bleeding after childbirth and in the treatment of migraine headaches. While the ergot alkaloids can be used clinically in the treatment of migraine headaches, in the two classes of hallucinogenic chemicals, indolamines including the ergoline LSD and phenylalkylamines, such as mescaline, the hallucinogens have not been used clinically for some time. Recently, interest has developed in the use of hallucinogens for the treatment of very specific medical problems. Psilocybin (Vollenweider and Kometer, 2010) and mescaline (Hermle et al., 1998; Heekeren et al., 2007) are undergoing clinical testing to determine the physiological effects of these hallucinogens and their potential use in relieving the anxiety associated with terminal cancer (Grob et al., 2010). Other ergot alkaloids are currently being examined for their possible treatment of cluster headaches (Sewell et al., 2006).

Alfred Hoffman, a synthetic chemist working for Sandoz pharmaceuticals, was interested in the chemistry of ergot alkaloids and first synthesized LSD-25 in 1938. The history of LSD is not long; however, it is very colorful (Hoffmann, 1979). LSD is a semi-synthetic substance that has lysergic acid as its parent compound. It has been a controversial drug almost from the beginning (Figure 9.1). Hoffman was attempting to synthesize a drug that was structurally similar to ergotamine, and he hoped it would act as a respiratory and circulatory stimulant. Testing showed no significant activity. In synthesizing a new batch of LSD, he was accidentally exposed, and Hoffman experienced the first "acid trip," still celebrated as "bicycle day" in Switzerland (Hoffman, 1980). Hoffman (1980) initially thought that LSD-25 had potential as a psychiatric drug, which would help patients "open-up." Hoffman realized that LSD was a potent hallucinogen; the medical community thought it was a wonder drug and a new research tool to be examined by pharmacologists over the next decade. Interest from other sectors of society developed, the Central Intelligence Agency (CIA) thought it might have potential for mind control, the British thought it might act as a truth serum, and the "hippie" generation saw it as a path to "spiritual enlightenment" and as a recreational drug (Hordern, 1968). It was quickly accepted by the "hippie" generation and rejected by the medical profession. Today, the primary medical use for LSD-25 is in the research laboratory where it has helped elucidate the role and function of 5-HT receptors. Timothy Leary and Richard Alpert were at Harvard University at the time LSD was discovered. Leary felt that LSD was a useful tool to expand one's mind and increase spiritual awareness. His contribution to the science of LSD was that he determined the median effective dose in adults for LSD, which is approximately 100 μg taken orally (The median effective dose (ED_{50}) is that dose which produces the desired effect in 50% of the population (Mosby's Medical Dictionary. 2009. 8th edn. Elsevier)).

The National Institute of Drug Abuse (NIDA) also became interested in hallucinogens and specifically LSD. A great deal of research was sponsored by NIDA, centered around an attempt to determine the mechanism of action of LSD, the neurotoxicity of hallucinogens and a determination of the lethal or toxic dose of LSD. In rats and humans a toxic/lethal dose was never determined. After more than 50 years of research on LSD, it is still not known what makes this compound so potent (Passie et al., 2008). It is, however, accepted that the hallucinogenic potency of either indolamines (LSD) or phenethylamine hallucinogens is highly correlated with the drugs affinity for the 5-HT$_2$ receptor (Glennon et al., 1984; Titeler et al., 1988). One question that should be asked is, what is a hallucination and how can it be studied in the laboratory animal?

WHAT IS A HALLUCINATION?

A hallucination can be defined as a visual, auditory, tactile, olfactory, or kinesthetic perception, which occurs in the absence of an external stimulus. A conscience experience of sound, taste, smell, or touch, all with no external input. It is not an illusion, which is a distortion of an external stimulus.

MECHANISM OF ACTION

The mechanism of action of LSD has been a challenge to determine. The pharmacology of LSD is very complex and even though it has been extensively studied the mechanism/s by which LSD exerts its effects are still not completely understood.

Behavioral models, using animals, are difficult to assess if one is testing a psychedelic drug. Even in monkeys, the behavior seen by a trained observer is difficult to quantify, when the behavior that is measured is a hallucination. Anden et al. (1968) were among the first to suggest that hallucinogens acted as a 5-HT agonist. In drug discrimination experiments, Glennon et al. (1983) demonstrated that hallucinogens might act primarily at 5-HT$_2$ receptors. In these studies rats were trained to discriminate between the phenethylamine hallucinogen 2,5-dimethoxy-4-methylamphetamine (DOM) and saline. The 5-HT$_2$ receptor antagonist, ketanserin, blocked the response, thereby implicating stimulation of the 5-HT$_{2A}$ receptor as a potential site of action for the production of hallucinations. These studies also suggested that the phenethylamine and the indolamine hallucinogens might share a common site of action. Glennon et al. (1984) linked the potency of a hallucinogen with its affinity for the 5-HT$_{2A}$ receptor. In other attempts to determine which receptor subtype produced the hallucinogenic response, several investigators reported that antagonists selective for the 5-HT$_{2A}$ receptor blocked the phenethylamine, as well as the indole hallucinogen more effectively than a 5-HT$_{2C}$ receptor antagonist (Pompeiano et al., 1994; Wright et al., 1995; Fiorella et al., 1995).

In behavioral studies, several unique responses have been identified that can be used in drug screening experiments (Halberstadt et al., 2009). It has been demonstrated that the "head twitch response" and the "ear scratch response" are specific responses to hallucinogenic drugs in the rodent. While these behavioral paradigms are useful for screening potential drug effects, it is difficult to project this behavior to human responses, but the predictive value is important. In other behavioral studies, the selective responses (i.e., head twitch and ear scratch responses) were abolished when LSD was given to 5-HT$_{2A}$ receptor knockout mice (Gonzalez-Maeso et al., 2007; Halberstadt et al., 2009), again implicating the 5-HT$_{2A}$ receptor in eliciting hallucinations.

Recent studies have demonstrated that LSD also produces an increase in the release of glutamate through stimulation of the 5-HT$_{2A}$ receptor (Aghajanian and Marek, 2000; Crawford et al., 2011). These findings suggest that the interaction between the 5-HT$_{2A}$ receptor and glutamate may be a necessary component of the "mechanism of action" of hallucinogenic drugs. (As can be seen in Figure 9.3.)

Passie et al. (2008) have suggested that hallucinogens may be producing a disinhibition in some systems as a possible mechanism of action. In the "Passie Hypothesis" it is necessary to accept that some 5-HT neurons must be inhibitory neurotransmitters in the *locus coeruleus* (LC). Therefore, when the activity of these 5-HT neurons is decreased, the activity of the subsequent neuron would be increased. This would not hold for all 5-HT

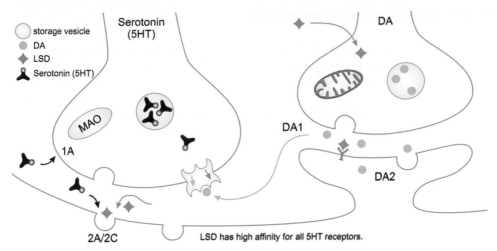

Figure 9.2   The serotonin neuron and the effects of lysergic acid diethylamide on this neuron.

neurons. As an example, the 5-HT$_3$ receptor is an excitatory ion channel receptor. Also, any subtype dependant on G protein coupling that produces an excitatory effect would be excluded from this generalization. Taking these exceptions into account, it may be possible to explain the mechanism of action of LSD and other hallucinogens as producing a "disinhibition" in some systems.

An examination of the 5-HT neuron (Figure 9.2 or revisit Chapter 2) reveals several obvious points for drug (LSD)/pre- or postsynaptic receptor interaction. These different drug–receptor interactions help define the mechanism of action of LSD. The primary actions of LSD on the 5-HT pre- and/or post-synaptic receptors are listed below. While there are also effects on other transmitter systems, it is generally agreed that the effects listed below contribute to the mechanism of action of LSD.

1. LSD acts as a partial agonist at the 5-HT$_{2A}$ receptor.
2. LSD acts as an agonist at the 5-HT$_{1A}$ receptor.
3. Stimulation of the 5-HT$_{1A}$ receptor produces a negative feedback, such that less 5-HT is released.
4. LSD competes at 5-HT 1, 2, 4, and 5 receptors with a very high affinity.
5. The amount of 5-HT at the receptor is reduced.
6. A 5-HT$_{2A}$ receptor antagonist can block the effect of LSD.
7. Activation of 5-HT$_{2A}$ receptors in the cortex, indirectly blocks response to glutamate via NMDA receptors.
8. LSD also acts at the DA D$_1$ and D$_2$ receptors.
9. Glutamate interacts with 5-HT neurons (Figure 9.3).

CLASSES OF HALLUCINOGENS

Over the years, attempts have been made to classify hallucinogens under different headings. Lewin categorized the group of drugs that we call hallucinogens as "phantastica" in the 1930s. In the 1960s he described the hallucinogens as "psychedelics" (mind viewing). Recently, because the hallucinogens produce an altered state of reality, possibly even a psychotic state, they are referred to as "psychotomimetic drugs." The categories listed below are based on the chemical structure of the hallucinogen. While there are many differences between the groups of compounds listed below, they all have one property in common; they produce some form of a hallucination (Katzung et al., 2009).

There are at least five categories of hallucinogens.

1. Lysergic acid derivatives, that is, LSD.
2. Phenylalkylamines, that is, mescaline, plant product, and methamphetamine or 3,4-methylenedioxy-N-methylamphetamine (MDMA), synthetic product.
3. Indolalkylamines, that is, psilocybin, plant product.
4. Indole derivative, ibogaine, plant product.
5. Glutamate NMDA receptor antagonists, receptor antagonists, phencyclidine, and ketamine.

PERIPHERAL AND CENTRAL EFFECTS OF LYSERGIC ACID DIETHYLAMIDE

The peripheral effects of LSD are relatively mild. The changes seen in the peripheral nervous system reflect stimulation of the sympathetic branch of the autonomic nervous system. In most human subjects, there is a slight increase in the heart rate and blood pressure. If there is a change in pupil size they tend to be dilated and potentially there is also an increase in body temperature (Table 9.1). The parasympathetic signs include salivation and possible nausea. Respiration tends to remain unchanged. There are some individuals that experience a marked bradycardia and hypotension, although this is rare (Passie et al., 2008).

The central effects of LSD are the predominant and the most subjective effects. LSD accentuates wherever you are mentally at the time it takes effect. Most LSD trips include both a pleasant and an unpleasant

Table 9.1   Physiological Side Effects of Lysergic Acid Diethylamide

An increase in blood pressure	Dizziness
An increase in heart rate	Tremors
Loss of appetite	Dry mouth
Sweating	Nausea

component. The drug effects are unpredictable and may vary with the amount ingested and the user's personality, mood, expectations, and surroundings (Hoffman, 1980; Passie et al., 2008).

The main effects, however, are emotional and sensory alterations and the user's emotions may shift rapidly through a range of fear to euphoria. Colors, smells, sounds, and other sensations are highly intensified and produce a phenomenon known as synesthesia. Not all "trips" produce synesthesia. However, then the hallucinations are of altered shapes and colors, and an increased sense of hearing. Hoffman said in his book "My Problem Child" that the furniture in his apartment was swirling around in circles.

Synesthesia is defined as *when a person hears colors and feels sounds*. An easy way to think of synesthesia is to think of hearing the Taiko drums (large Japanese drums), where you can actually feel the sound in your chest.

There are also alterations in mood during an LSD trip. The mood of the user can start very happy and rapidly shift to sad or irritable. Occasionally the user will even experience panic attacks. There is a distorted sense of time and feelings like one is in a dream. Hoffman noted that he had difficulty speaking and expressing his thoughts on the day that he first used LSD (Hoffman, 1980).

LONG-TERM EFFECTS OF LYSERGIC ACID DIETHYLAMIDE

Psychosis

There have been no reported deaths from LSD; this, however, does not mean that there are no serious side effects. There are two long-term effects that can occur from frequent LSD use: the first, a persistent psychosis that resembles a type of paranoid schizophrenia and paranoid delusions. This psychosis can require hospitalization. The psychosis may include a distortion or disorganization of a person's capacity to recognize reality, think rationally, or communicate with others (Iversen et al., 2009). Some users also experience mood swings that can be dramatic, ranging from mania to profound depression and then to vivid hallucinations. In some cases, the psychosis-type reaction appears to be short lived. However, in many cases the induced psychosis is chronic and long lasting. It is difficult to determine if LSD simply triggers an underlying condition or weakened state, or if it is the cause of the psychosis.

Flashbacks

The second long-term effect is "flashbacks" often and interchangeably referred to as hallucination persisting perception disorder (HPPD). Flashbacks are a psychological phenomenon where one experiences some of the subjective effects of LSD, even after the drug is no longer present in the system. In some cases this occurs several days after the last dose of LSD, and may continue to recur for many years after the last use of LSD (Halpern and Pope, 2003). It is not known what stimulus precipitates the flashback. The flashback tends to be relatively mild and short lived (some lasting only for seconds), but they can incorporate both negative and positive aspects of the LSD trip. While it is difficult to determine what triggers the flashback, they can be triggered by alcohol, stress, or something as simple as a sound or a smell (Lerner et al., 2002).

There is no explanation as to why flashbacks occur; however, they do appear to be linked to the use of LSD. While 70% of LSD users do not report experiencing flashbacks, many of those who have, tend to be psychiatric patients (Abrahart, 1998; Naditch and Fenwick, 1977).

Flashbacks are not recognized as a medical disease in the United States; however, hallucinogen persisting perception disorder (HPPD) is a recognized syndrome. HPPD is described in the DSM-IV as a syndrome in which LSD-like visual changes occur. The visual changes are not brief and temporary in nature, but rather cause extreme distress and psychological impairment. HPPD is entirely visual. It has been suggested that HPPD is a form of post-traumatic stress disorder and as such is in no way related to the use of LSD. There are several important differences between "flashbacks" and HPPD. (1) Duration; flashback occurs for a very short period of time, while HPPD can be long lasting. (2) The emotional feelings produced by flashbacks are not necessarily negative, while HPPD tends to produce negative feelings (Lerner et al., 2002). (3) Flashbacks are not listed in the DSM-IV, and therefore not considered a medical disorder to be treated. However, flashbacks are defined by the WHO International Classification of Diseases, Version 10 (ICD-10) as a very short re-experiencing of a past drug trip that may spontaneously occur or be self-induced when the hallucinations were positive.

TOXICITY AND TOLERANCE

Tolerance develops fairly quickly to LSD, such that increasingly larger doses are required to produce the same effect if used daily. The tolerance dissipates after roughly 1 week, therefore, the same dose can be used weekly.

A cross-tolerance also occurs to other hallucinogens such as psilocybin and mescaline (Passie et al., 2008). These drugs can be used interchangeably, although LSD is far more potent. The cross-tolerance does not extend to the hallucinogens from any of the non-indole classifications, namely amphetamine, phencyclidine (PCP), or marijuana.

Routes of Administration

Of the plant-based hallucinogens, LSD is the most potent mood-altering drug known today (Glennon et al., 1984; Glennon and Titeler, 1986). Oral doses, as low as 25–30 μg can produce effects that last for 6–12 hours. The methods used to distribute the drug are varied, but the most common way consisted of crushing the crystals into a powder, dissolving the powder in water and adding paper to the water. This solution was then absorbed by a piece of paper, this form of LSD was known as "blotter acid." Others mixed the powder with a binding agent, and made small tablets that were called "microdots." At one Grateful Dead concert in the 1960s, Ken Kesey added a microdot to each concert ticket. He was working at a VA Hospital and managed to take LSD while working. It was at this time that he wrote, "One Flew Over The Cuckoo's Nest."

PHARMACOKINETICS

The effects of LSD last for approximately 6–12 hours depending on the dose taken. The elimination half-life for LSD has been reported to be 175 minutes (Aghajanian et al., 1964). More recent data, (Papac and Foltz, 1990) found a half-life of 5.1 hours, with the peak plasma levels occurring at 3 hours after ingestion of LSD.

A lethal dose has never been found in laboratory animals or humans.

CANDY FLIPPING

The practice of taking 3,4-methylenedioxy-N-methylamphetamine (MDMA) and LSD together to enhance the "overall effect" was first started in the 1990s at rave parties in California (Schechter, 1998). These parties usually occurred in the desert in California and were somewhat similar to Woodstock, without the live rock groups. This particular combination of drugs, MDMA in combination with LSD was called "candy flipping" on the street. Candy flipping was thought to improve the experience that was produced from taking LSD alone. MDMA added euphoria and the "good feelings" that were missing from an LSD trip. While MDMA was producing a feeling of euphoria, LSD made the euphoric feeling seem more intense. LSD altered one's mental function, while MDMA made everything seem to move faster. A comparison of the multiple sites of action of MDMA and 5-HT can be found in Table 9.2.

While these two drugs have different mechanisms of action, their differences seem to compliment and potentiate the effects of the other drug. Taken in combination, LSD (acting as a partial agonist at the 5-HT$_{2A}$ receptor) potentiates the neurotoxic effects of MDMA, thus supporting the model of Sprague and Nichols (1995). This hypothesis was confirmed and extended by Armstrong (2002) where he extends the action of the two drugs to include actions on glutamate and GABA. The neurotoxic actions of MDMA and LSD occur most commonly in the following regions. See Figure 9.3 for the possible actions of MDMA and LSD.

Table 9.2   A Comparison of the Sites of Action of Lysergic Acid Diethylamide (LSD) and 3,4-methylenedioxy-*N*-methylamphetamine (MDMA)

MDMA	LSD
Releases dopamine and serotonin	Is an agonist at the D_1 receptor
Is an agonist at the 5-HT_2 receptor	Is a partial agonist at the 5-HT_{2A} receptor
Is a phenethylamine	Is an indole amine
MDMA degeneration at axons and dendrites	
Both are potentially neurotoxic in animals and humans	
Both alter the release of glutamate	

MDMA produces degeneration at the nerve ending in the:

1. Raphe nucleus
2. Cortex
3. Neostriatum
4. Hippocampus

The neurotoxic effect produces a loss of both axons and dendrites. In animal studies the neurotoxic effect found in the hippocampus produced anterograde amnesia, not retrograde amnesia. In humans, the effect of an adult dose (~100 mg) can produce depression, sleep disturbance, and new memories are not stored.

To examine the potentially altered toxicity when MDMA and LSD are taken simultaneously, one might first look at which areas of the brain contain both DA and 5-HT neurons in close proximity to each other. One area is the hippocampus. Studies have demonstrated that there is degeneration of 5-HT nerve endings in the hippocampus after MDMA (Armstrong, 2002). Other investigators have also demonstrated that there is a linear relation between DA release and 5-HT terminal damage (Nash and Nichols, 1991) and pretreatment with a DA synthesis inhibitor protects against 5-HT terminal damage (Stone et al., 1988). When DA is taken up into the 5-HT terminals, free radicals are formed, potentially leading to terminal dying. In humans, this could lead to depression and a decrease in learning and memory. It was also demonstrated that if one administered fluoxetine (Prozac) prior to administration of MDMA, the neurotoxicity did not occur or the effects of MDMA were blocked (Sprague and Nichols, 1995). If the nerve was only injured, it was demonstrated that the nerve terminals grew back; however, the new synapses were not the same. When the terminals are not in the same place, they could make abnormal connections and possibly produce abnormal responses.

While the mechanisms involved in the use of MDMA and LSD together are not precisely known, there are several reasoned hypotheses. One possible neurochemical response to this drug combination is shown in

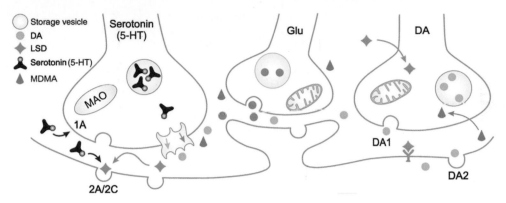

Storage vesicle
DA
LSD
Serotonin (5-HT)
MDMA

Serotonin
(5-HT)

MAO

1A

2A/2C

Glu

DA

DA1

DA2

Figure 9.3   Combination of 3,4-methylenedioxy-*N*-methylamphetamine and lysergic acid diethylamide, that is, candy flipping.

Figure 9.3. In this scenario both 5-HT and DA are released from their respective neurons. During the reuptake of 5-HT, the transporter also takes up DA. This is not an unreasonable hypothesis, as it has long been known that the 5-HT terminals will take up and release DA (Butcher et al., 1970). The DA in the 5-HT terminal may increase the concentration of free radicals thus producing neural degeneration (Levitt et al., 1982; Sprague and Nichols, 1995). One cannot help but wonder if DA is released from the 5-HT terminal, by whatever means, does it act like DA, or like 5-HT at the receptor, or is the response altered in some other way? A second mechanism would involve the increased release of glutamate (See Figure 9.3). Glutamate undoubtedly plays a role in the effects obtained by the MDMA + LSD drug combination. However, it is not known if it simply increases neurotoxicity (Parrott, 2012) or if it also provides enhanced excitatory stimulation (Schechter, 1998). Both MDMA (via DA receptors) and LSD (via 5-HT$_{2A}$ receptors) increase the release of glutamate and enhance the transmission of glutamate in the prefrontal cortex (Aghajanian and Marek, 2000). In a recent study, Moreno and colleagues (2011) suggested that the metabotropic glutamate receptor 2/3 (mgluR2), in fact modulated the response of the LSD-activated 5-HT$_{2A}$ receptor. These authors concluded that the 5-HT$_{2A}$ receptor and the mGluR2 receptor formed a necessary complex in the production of responses that are produced by hallucinogens (Moreno et al., 2011).

In summary, candy flipping or the addition of MDMA to LSD may reduce or even eliminate the possibility of a "bad trip"; however, and more importantly, it increases the possibility of free radical damage and neuronal cell death. The mechanisms of this drug interaction are yet to be completely defined.

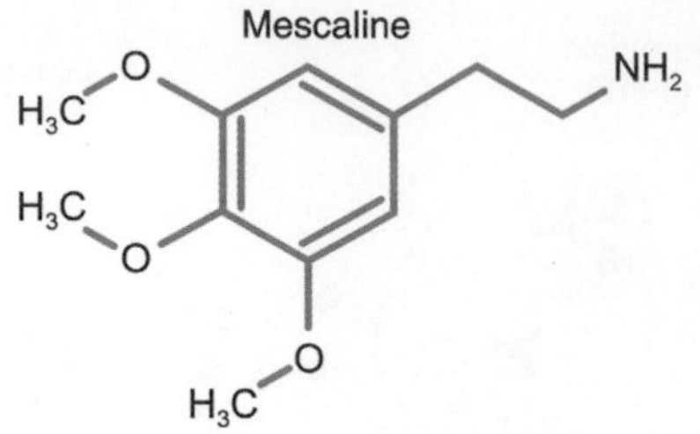

Figure 9.4   Structural formula for mescaline (3,4,5 trimethoxyphenethylamine).

MESCALINE (PEYOTE)

Mescaline is the active ingredient in the San Pedro cactus and the Peyote cactus (Figure 9.4). The buds, or "heads" of the cactus are removed and eaten, or they are boiled in water and drunk as a type of tea. Peyote use dates back to 300 BC and has been used by the Aztecs, Toltecs, and Chichimecas in religious ceremonies. Peyote is still used by Northern Mexican tribes and Southwest Plains Indian tribes in their religious ceremonies. By the 1900s the use of peyote had spread north to the United States, and was used by other Indian tribes in ceremonies. The Comprehensive Drug Abuse Prevention and Control Act made the use of peyote illegal in 1970. Peyote is illegal in most countries today, and even possession of, or growing the cactus, is now illegal in many countries.

MECHANISM OF ACTION

The mechanism of action of mescaline appears to be very similar to that of LSD, namely it is a partial agonist at the 5-HT$_{2A}$ receptor (Nichols, 2004; Beique et al., 2007). Mescaline also stimulates dopamine receptors, either by releasing dopamine or as a receptor agonist.

CENTRAL AND PERIPHERAL NERVOUS SYSTEM EFFECTS

Although weaker than LSD, the effects of mescaline are similar. Mescaline does produce an altered sense of self and an altered sense of time. Thinking processes become more abstract and synesthesia can also occur with mescaline as it does with LSD. The hallucinations that are experienced with mescaline are not true hallucinations, but rather altered images of the existing objects or sounds that the user sees and hears. Colors and sounds are more pronounced, almost appearing brilliant in their intensity. The effect is not a hallucination in that real objects are seen, not imaginary objects or sounds (Halberstadt and Geyer, 2011).

Mescaline also produces an increase in sympathetic arousal, such that the peripheral nervous system is stimulated. After approximately 1–2 hours, the user experiences an increase in respiration, heart rate, and blood pressure. The increase in sympathetic stimulation may last anywhere from 12–18 hours.

PHARMACOKINETICS

Tolerance to mescaline does develop with repeated use. The developed tolerance only lasts for a few days, or possibly a week. A cross-tolerance with other drugs in this category, that is, LSD, psilocybin, does occur. This cross-tolerance may be a result of a similar mechanism of action. Cross-tolerance does not develop between mescaline and THC.

The half-life of mescaline is ~6–8 hours, although there is a controversy as to the route of metabolism. Some studies suggest that mescaline is excreted unchanged in urine, while others report that it is metabolized by monoamine oxidase (MAO) and excreted as the carboxylic acid (Wu et al., 1997).

Review Questions

1. Discuss the effects of LSD as a partial agonist at the 5-HT$_{2A}$ receptor.
2. What are the classes of hallucinogens? Do PCP and ketamine fit into this classification?
3. Discuss the addictive potential of LSD.
4. Why do flashbacks occur?
5. Describe synesthesia.

REFERENCES AND ADDITIONAL READING

Abrahart D. 1998. A critical review of theories and research concerning lysergic acid diethylamide (LSD) and mental health. (http://www.maps.org/research/abrahart.html#chp1, accessed on July 25, 2012.)

Aghajanian GK, Bing OH. 1964. Persistence of lysergic acid diethylamide in the plasma of human subjects. *Clin. Pharmacol. Ther.* 5: 611–614.

Aghajanian GK, Marek GJ. 2000. Serotonin model of schizophrenia: emerging role of glutamate mechanisms. *Brain Res. Rev.* 31:302–312.

Anden NE, Corrodi H, Fuxe K. 1968. Evidence for a central 5-hydroxytryptamine receptor stimulation by lysergic acid diethylamide or bufotenin. *Br. J. Pharmacol.* 34:1–7.

Armstrong B. 2002. The use of Neuropsychopharmacological Experimental Methods in Elucidating the Relationship Between Serotonin and Dopamine in the Brain (PhD Dissertation, University of California, California, LA).

Beique JC, Imad M, Mladenovic, L, Gingrich, JA, Andrade R. 2007. Mechanism of the 5-hydroxytryptamine 2A receptor-mediated facilitation of synaptic activity in prefrontal cortex. *Proc. Natl. Acad. Sci. U.S.A.* 104:9870–9875.

Butcher L, Engel J, Fuxe K. 1970. L-dopa induced changes in central monoamine neurons after peripheral decarboxylase inhibition. *J. Pharm. Pharmacol.* 22:313–316.

Crawford LK, Craige CP, Beck SG. 2011. Glutamatergic input is selectively increased in dorsal raphe subfield 5-HT neurons: role of morphology, topography and selective innervation. *Eur. J. Neurosci.* 34:1794–1806.

Fiorella D, Rabin RA, Winter JC. 1995. The role of the 5-HT2A and 5-HT2C receptors in the stimulus effects of hallucinogenic drugs. I: Antagonist correlation analysis. *Psychopharmacol.* 121:347–356.

Glennon RA, Titeler M. 1986. Structure-activity relationships and mechanism of action of hallucinogenic agents based on drug discrimination and radioligand binding studies. *Psychopharmacol. Bull.* 22:953–958.

Glennon RA, Titeler M, McKenney JD. 1984. Evidence for 5-HT2 involvement in the mechanisms of action of hallucinogenic agents. *Life Sci.* 35:2505–2511.

Glennon RA, Young R, Rosecrans JA. 1983. Antagonism of the effects of the hallucinogen DOM and the purported 5-HT agonist quipazine by 5-HT2 antagonists. *Eur. J. Pharmacol.* 91: 189–96.

Gonzalez-Maeso J, Weisstaub NV, Zhou M, et al. 2007. Hallucinogens recruit specific cortical 5-HT$_{2A}$ receptor-mediated signaling pathways to affect behavior. *Neuron.* 53:439–452.

Grob CS, Danforth AL, Chopra GS, Hagerty M, McKay CR, Halberstadt AL, Greer GR. 2010. Pilot study of psilocybin treatment for anxiety in patients with advanced-stage cancer. *Arch. Gen. Psychiatry.* 68:71–78.

Halberstadt AL, Geyer MA. 2011. Multiple receptors contribute to the behavioral effects of indoleamine hallucinogens. *Neuropharmacol.* 61:364–381.

Halberstadt AL, van der Heijden I, Ruderman MA, et al. 2009. 5-HT 2A and 5-HT2C receptors exert opposing effects on locomotor activity in mice. *Neuropsychopharmacology.* 34:1958–1967.

Halpern JH, Pope HG Jr. 2003. Hallucinogen persisting perception disorder: what do we know after 50 years? *Drug Alcohol Depend.* 69:109–119.

Heekeren K, Neukirch A, Dauman J, et al. 2007. Prepulse inhibition of the startle reflex and its attentional modulation in human models of psychosis. *J. Psychopharmacol.* 21:312–320.

Hermle L, Goupoulis-Mayfrank E, Spitzer M. 1998. Blood flow and cerebral laterality in the mescaline model of psychosis. *Pharmacopsychiatry. Suppl.* 2085–2091.

Hoffman A. 1979. Hallucinogens, shamanism and modern life. *J. Psychedetic Drugs.* 11:1–23.

Hoffman A. 1980. *LSD: My Problem Child*. McGraw Hill, New York.

Hordern A. 1968. Psychopharmacology: some historical considerations. In: Joyce CRB (ed), *Psychopharmacology: Dimensions and Perspectives*. JB Lippincott, Philadelphia.

Iversen LL, Iversen SD, Bloom FE, Roth RH. 2009. *Introduction to Neuropsychopharmacology*. Oxford University Press, New York.

Katzung BG, Masters SB, Trevor AJ. 2009. *Basic and Clinical Pharmacology. Drugs of Abuse*. McGraw Hill Medical, New York.

Lee MR. 2010. The history of ergot of rye (Claviceps purpurea) III: 1940–80. *J. R. Coll. Physicians Edinb.* 40:77–80.

Lerner AG, Gelkopf M, Skladman I, et al. 2002. Flashback and Hallucinogen persisting perception disorder: clinical aspects and pharmacological treatment approach. *Isr. J. Psychiatry Relat. Sci.* 39:92–99.

Levitt P, Pintar JE, Breakfield XO. 1982. Immunocytochemical demonstration of monoamine oxidase-B in brain astrocytes and serotonergic neurons. *Proc. Natl. Acad. Sci. USA.* 79:6385–6389.

Moreno JL, Holloway T, Albizu L, Sealfon SC, Gonzalez-Maeso J. 2011. Metabotropic glutamate mGlu2 receptor is necessary for the pharmacological and behavioural effects induced by hallucinogenic 5-HT2A receptor agonists. *Neurosci. Lett.* 493:76–79.

Naditch MP, Fenwick S. 1977. LSD flashbacks and ego functioning. *J. Abnormal Psych.* 86: 352–359.

Nash JF, Nicholls DE. 1991. Microdialysis studies of MDMA and structurally related analogues. *Eur. J. Pharm.* 200:53–58.

Nichols DE. 2004. Hallucinogens. *Pharmacol. Ther.* 101: 131–181.

Papac DI, Foltz RL. 1990. Measurement of lysergic acid diethylamide (LSD) in human plasma by gas chromatography/negative ion chemical ionization mass spectrometry. *J. Anal. Toxicol.* 14:189–190.

Parrott AC. 2012. MDMA and 5-HT neurotoxicity: the empirical evidence for its adverse effects in humans-no need for translation. *Br. J. Pharmacol.* 166:1518–1520.

Passie T, Halpern JH, Stichtenoth DO, Emrich HM, Hintzen A. 2008. The pharmacology of lysergic acid diethyl amine: a Review. *CNS Neurosci. Ther.* 14:295–314.

Pompeiano M, Palacios JM, Mengod G. 1994. Distribution of the serotonin 5-HT2 receptor family mRNAs: comparison between 5-HT2A and 5-HT2C receptors. *Brain Res. Mol. Brain Res.* 23:163–78.

Schechter MD. 1998. "Candyflipping": synergistic discriminative effect of LSD and MDMA. *Eur. J. Pharmacol.* 341:131–134.

Schultz RE, Hoffman A. 1980. *Plants of the Gods*. McGraw-Hill, New York.

Sewell RA, Halpern JH, Pope HG Jr. 2006. Response of cluster headache to psilocybin and LSD. *Neurology.* 66:1920–1922.

Sprague JE, Nichols DE. 1995. The monoamine oxidase-B inhibitor L-deprenyl protects against MDMA-induced lipid peroxidation and long-term serotonergic deficits. *J. Pharm. Exp. Ther.* 273:667–673.

Stone DM, Johnson M, Hanson GR, Gibb JW. 1988. Role of endogenous dopamine in the central serotonergic deficits induced by MDMA. *J. Pharm. Exp. Ther.* 247:79–87.

Titeler M, Lyon RA, Glennon RA. 1988. Radioligand binding evidence implicates the brain 5-HT$_2$ receptor as a site of action for LSD and phenylisopropylamine hallucinogens. *Psychopharmacol.* 94:213–216.

Vollenweider FX, Kometer M. 2010. The neurobiology of psychedelic drugs: implications for mood disorders. *Nat. Rev. Neurosci.* 11:624–651.

Wright DE, Seroogy KB, Lundgren KH, Davis BM, Jennes L. 1995. Comparative localization of serotonin 1A, 1C, and 2 receptor subtype mRNAs in rat brain. *J. Comp. Neurol.* 351:357–373.

Wu D, Otton SV, Inaba T, Kalow W, Sellers EM. 1997. Interaction of amphetamine analogs with human liver CYP2D6. *Biochem. Pharmacol.* 53:1605–1612.

10 Marijuana

Learning Objectives

The student will learn:

1. The potential mechanism of action of marijuana (delta-9-tetrahydrocannabinol or THC).
2. The primary effects of THC in the central nervous system.
3. The primary effects of THC in the peripheral nervous system.
4. Clinical uses for THC.
5. Side effects of chronic use of THC.
6. The side effects of abruptly stopping marijuana use.

The earliest recorded history of *Cannabis* use was in 2737 BC. The Chinese emperor, Shen Nung, wrote in a pharmacy book about the medicinal use of *Cannabis* for female weakness, rheumatism, malaria, constipation, and absent-mindedness. Social use spread to North Africa and the Muslim world by 1000 AD and legends developed around the use of *Cannabis* by a religious cult that committed political murders. The cult was called the "hashishiyya" and this name is the basis of the English word, assassin.

Over the centuries tales of mystery and intrigue have been part of the "culture" of *Cannabis* and hashish. From Marco Polo and tales from The Arabian Nights, to Napoleon's campaign in Egypt which caused soldiers to become familiar with the use of hashish. Napoleon forbid the use of hashish among his soldiers, but the use was still very high. It was rumored that they also returned home with a supply of hashish. This was the introduction of hashish to Europe and the use of hashish can be found in many French novels.

Cannabis came to the Americas, but the use of the plant by early colonists seemed to be primarily for the making of hemp. *Cannabis* was grown even by president George Washington. By the twentieth century limited recreational use of marijuana could also be found in the United States. Public concern was not aroused, as the use was rather limited. However, the police departments started to associate violent crimes with marijuana use.

Drugs of Abuse: Pharmacology and Molecular Mechanisms, First Edition. Sherrel G. Howard.
© 2014 John Wiley & Sons, Inc. Published 2014 by John Wiley & Sons, Inc.

Newspaper articles and magazines so exaggerated the use of marijuana that the Federal Bureau of Narcotics held congressional hearings, resulting in laws that regulated the use, sale, or possession of marijuana. Movies such as "Reefer Madness" helped build the case for the dangers of marijuana use. Over the years, this perception has changed. While there is evidence that marijuana, as any other recreational drug, is potentially addictive, several states in the Union, for example, Washington and Colorado have recently passed laws that legalize marijuana use and many more states have passed laws that decriminalize its use, at least for medical purposes. In other states there is continuing discussion about legalization, due to the undeniable benefits that marijuana provides for patients with chronic pain, HIV, chemotherapy-induced nausea, multiple sclerosis, and other neurodegenerative diseases.

Today, in the United States, marijuana is the most commonly used illicit drug (Sofuoglu et al., 2010; SAMHSA, 2008). A National Survey on Drug Use and Health (2003) reported that over 40% of the American population aged 12 and older had tried marijuana at least once and of the 2–3 million currently using marijuana, one in 12 will become dependent (Wagner and Anthony, 2002). SAMHSA (2008) reported an increase in marijuana users from 14.5 million to 18.1 million.

By 2010, more than 29 millions Americans (11.5%) aged 12 and older reported using marijuana within the past year, a significant increase over rates reported each year from 2002 to 2008 (SAMHSA, 2010). According to NIDA's Monitoring the Future study of eighth, tenth, and twelfth graders, a consistent decline in marijuana use began in the mid-1990s and continued into the early 2000s. But in the past few years this trend has reversed with 5-year trends showing significant increases among tenth and twelfth graders for daily, current, and past year use. This year, 12.5% of eighth graders, 28.8% of tenth graders, and 36.4% of twelfth graders reported past-year marijuana use. This year's survey also reported the use of synthetic marijuana, also known as K2 or "Spice" among high school seniors (Atwood et al., 2010).

SYNTHESIS OF MARIJUANA

Marijuana is biosynthesized by the plant *Cannabis sativa*, the hemp plant. The active ingredient in marijuana is delta-9-tetrahydrocannabinol (THC), which is also the active ingredient in hashish. Figure 10.1 shows the structural formula for marijuana.

The biosynthetic pathway is:

Cannabindiol (CBD) → delta-9-tetrahydrocannabinol (THC) → Cannabinol (CBN).

By measuring the proportion of these components;

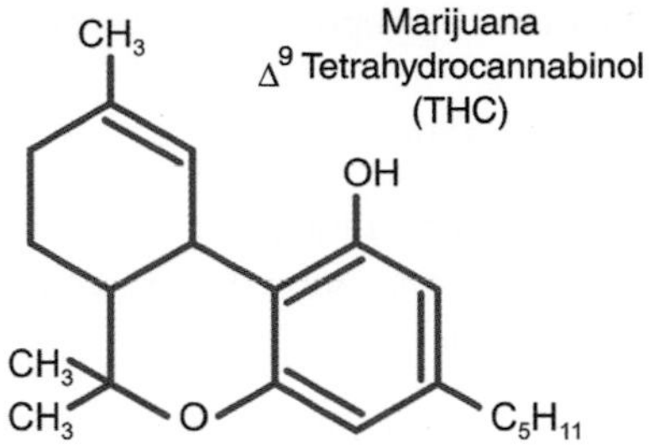

CH₃

Marijuana
Δ⁹ Tetrahydrocannabinol
(THC)

Figure 10.1   Structural formula for delta-9-tetrahydrocannabinol.

Percentage of THC/plant ~1%
In genetically altered plants:
Percentage of THC/plant ~4-6%

Other cannabinoids in the hemp plant include cannabidiol (CBD) and cannabinol (CBN) as shown above. Although CBD displays no particular affinity for the CB1 receptors, it can act as an indirect antagonist of cannabinoid agonists, with anxiolytic effects. It is also a 5-HT1A receptor agonist, as well as an allosteric modulator of μ and δ opioid receptors.

MECHANISM OF ACTION OF DELTA-9-TETRAHYDROCANNABINOL

THC exerts its primary effects by activating or inhibiting the cannabinoid receptors, CB1 and CB2. Both of these receptors are G-protein linked receptors (Wilson and Nicoll, 2002).

The CB1 receptors are located throughout the brain and are primarily located presynaptically on both excitatory and inhibitory nerve terminals. For example, when stimulation of the CB1 receptor produces presynaptic inhibition at a GABA nerve terminal, then THC will produce a disinhibition of dopamine neurons, primarily by presynaptic inhibition of GABA release. This disinhibition will produce an increase in the release of dopamine.

The CB2 receptors are located predominantly in the peripheral nervous system. In the brain they occur mainly in microglia. They are also associated with the immune system.

THC also modulates dopaminergic transmission via the CB1 receptor. Recent data suggests that this modulation is primarily through indirect mechanisms (Fitzgerald et al., 2012; Svensson, 2000); however, it has also been suggested that there is a direct effect on the DA D_1 receptor by enhancing the frequency of postsynaptic currents, which are excitatory and on the DA D_2 receptor by contributing to D_2 receptor inhibition (Andre et al., 2010).

Cannabinoid receptors are typical members of the G-protein coupled receptors.

They are as follows:

1. Linked to inhibition of adenylate cyclase
2. The receptor is coupled to K$^+$ channel activation
3. Ca^{++} channel inhibition

Therefore, one would predict an inhibitory effect on neurotransmitter release or a disinhibition on a secondary neuron. These effects are similar to opioids, discussed in Chapter 8.

NEUROANATOMICAL DISTRIBUTION

The distribution of CB1 receptors in the brain corresponds to the primary pharmacological effects of THC.

1. Hippocampus, memory impairment
2. Cerebellum, basal ganglia, motor disturbance
3. Mesolimbic dopamine (DA), pathway reward
4. Ventral tegmental area (VTA), pain

PERIPHERAL AND CENTRAL EFFECTS OF DELTA-9-TETRAHYDROCANNABINOL

THC acts primarily in the central nervous system, producing a psychotomimetic or depressant effect via the CB1 receptor.

The effects in the periphery are mild, but still noticeable. In the periphery, CB2 receptors are located mainly in the lymphoid system and may account for the inhibitory effects of THC on the immune function. Other milder effects can include tachycardia, vasodilation, and bronchodilation (Table 10.1).

THC exerts its primary effects in the central nervous system (CNS) as well as on the cardiovascular system. In humans, THC produces an effect on mood, motor coordination, memory, cognition, sense of time, and a sense of euphoria. The most common effects found in humans are listed below.

Main Effects in Humans

1. Feelings of relaxation similar to ethanol, but with no feelings of aggression.
2. Feelings of sharpened sensory awareness with respect to sound and sights. Sounds are more intense.
3. Balance is affected even at low doses of THC.

4. At moderate-to-high doses, simple motor tasks can be impaired, as
    well as memory. Driving is significantly impaired, as is information
    processing after one or two cigarettes.

Table 10.1   Central and Peripheral Effects of THC

1. Time passes slowly
2. Decrease in short-term memory
3. A feeling of confidence, but performance does not reflect this
4. Impaired motor coordination, driving ability
5. Catalepsy
6. Analgesia
7. Antiemetic action
8. Increased appetite

Peripheral Effects

1. Tachycardia (this can be blocked)
2. Vasodilation (most pronounced in the conjunctiva of the eye; producing the
    blood-shot eye look)
3. Decreased intraocular pressure
4. Bronchodilation

There are many effects that are reported by marijuana smokers that occur frequently, but not on all occasions. These include hunger, dry mouth,
improved hearing, dramatic visual images, and so on, but surprisingly
marijuana tends to decrease empathy with others and dialogues are impaired or nonexistent. The perception of time is altered when smoking
marijuana and this seems to be a consistent effect with all smokers.

At high doses, marijuana can produce hallucinations, paranoia, and
confused and disorganized thought. Instead of the feelings of euphoria experienced with moderate doses of THC, the euphoria can be replaced with
anxiety. With very high doses, a toxic psychosis and hallucinations can occur. According to Perez-Reyes (Perez-Reyes et al., 1982) use of marijuana
can precipitate "flashbacks" in former users of lysergic acid diethylamide
(LSD).

CLINICAL USES FOR DELTA-9-TETRAHYDROCANNABINOL

There are several therapeutic applications for THC or a synthetic analog
of THC. The most common uses are listed below; however, recent studies have also suggested that synthetic analogs of THC may be useful as
analgesics and also as anticonvulsants.

1. Reduces intraocular pressure in glaucoma patients
2. Bronchial pain
3. Anti-emetic action

Some medicaments derived from cannabis include dronabinol and Sativex. Dronabinol, sold as Marinol, is an isomer of THC. It is administered orally so that one does have to deal with the problem of first pass metabolism. However, most of the metabolites that are produced are active metabolites. Dronabinol has been approved by the US Food and Drug Administration(US FDA) for the treatment of anorexia in AIDS patients and to treat nausea and vomiting in patients undergoing chemotherapy. Sativex, which contains both THC and CBD, is a mouth spray used by multiple sclerosis patients to relieve neuropathic pain and spasticity.

CENTRAL NERVOUS SYSTEM EFFECTS OF A CB1 RECEPTOR ANTAGONIST

Anandamide is one of the first endogenous cannabinoid compounds discovered. It is derived from arachidonic acid. Since the discovery of anandamide, several CB1 antagonists, such as Rimonabant (SR141716A) have been developed that produce effects opposite to those obtained from an agonist, such as the following.

1. Increase in locomotor activity
2. Improved short-term memory
3. Increase in neurotransmitter release

These and many other studies led to the development of several marijuana analogs (Howlett et al., 1990).

CHRONIC AND LONG-TERM USE OF MARIJUANA

Attitudes toward smoking marijuana have ranged from unfounded fear to unquestioning acceptance. But the fact remains that the long-term chronic use of marijuana has numerous adverse effects. Among the many adverse effects of long-term use of marijuana are a negative effect on pulmonary function and the bronchial epithelium resulting in bronchitis or asthma, development of the "amotivational syndrome" which consists of apathy, impaired judgment, concentration, and memory, loss of interest in appearance, and lack of interest in conventional goals (Fehr and Kalant, 1983; Jones, 1983). It should be noted that the tar that is produced by the pyrolysis (smoking) of marijuana is more carcinogenic to man and animals than that derived from tobacco (Petersen, 1980). While there is no evidence that any of these changes are due to damages in the brain, nerves or vessels. It is possible permanent changes in personality or mood can occur from the continued use of Marijuana. Table 10.2 shows alterations due to chronic use of marijuana.

Table 10.2   Chronic Users of Marijuana
Exhibit the Following Symptoms

Apathy
Impairment of judgment
Impairment of concentration
Impairment of short-term memory
Loss of interest in appearance
Loss of interest in goals

Marijuana is thought to produce an amotivational syndrome. Of course there are always arguments in favor of marijuana, suggesting that none of these behaviors can be clearly attributed to marijuana alone.

Endocrine Changes

Studies on the effect of chronic long-term use of THC on human sexual function have obtained conflicting results. There are reports of a decrease in serum testosterone and a decrease in spermatogenesis, which is reversible. In women, anovulatory cycles as well as a decrease in follicle stimulating hormone (FSH) and luteinizing hormone (LH) have also been reported. In studies using male and female monkeys, it has been demonstrated that the hypothalamic–pituitary axis is inhibited. These data could explain some alterations in the endocrine function. When exposed to THC during pregnancy (in humans and animals) the offspring exhibits deficits in learning and response to stimuli (Fehr and Kalant, 1983). In a more recent study, DiNieri and coworkers (2011) have demonstrated that prenatal exposure to cannabis decreased expression of the DA D_2 receptor mRNA in the human ventral striatum/nucleus accumbens. Repeating the studies in rats produced the same results, which could then be extended to determine if any deficit was found in the adult animal. Their results demonstrated that regulation of the D_2 receptor was altered and that the alteration was not reversible. The authors concluded that this permanent alteration in the D_2 receptor could contribute to an increased sensitivity to opiates in adulthood (DiNieri et al., 2011).

ROUTE OF ADMINISTRATION AND ABSORPTION OF DELTA-9-TETRAHYDROCANNABINOL

The preferred route of marijuana administration is by smoking; however, it is also taken orally and via some type of vaporizer. Because of the high lipid solubility of THC, it is trapped in the lining of the lungs and rapidly absorbed into the system. Dried leaves, stems, and flowers can be easily hand-rolled into "joints" and smoked. Marijuana can also be smoked in water pipes or "bongs" or in "blunts" where a cigar is cut open and the tobacco replaced with marijuana. If taken orally, either mixed in food or combined with another drug in a tea, the rate of absorption is more variable and the duration of action is longer.

Absorption

The absorption of marijuana occurs very quickly reaching peak concentrations in plasma in less than 10 minutes. The total duration of action of THC is approximately 2–3 hours. Marijuana is very lipophilic, and approximately 60% of marijuana is absorbed. The other 40% is metabolized at a variable rate depending on the user.

Chronic use of THC increases the rate of metabolism of cannabinoids over that of non-smokers. The rate of metabolism of barbiturates and alcohol is also altered in chronic THC users.

TOLERANCE, ADDICTION, AND PHYSICAL DEPENDENCE

Tolerance does develop to some of the effects of marijuana. In animal studies, it has been demonstrated that a tolerance develops to the decrease in temperature found after marijuana exposure as well as some of the behavioral effects.

In Humans

Experienced users show less impairment of perceptual and motor functions. The increase in heart rate in experienced users is not as great as that found in the inexperienced user. This increase in heart rate is still problematic as marijuana reduces the oxygen-carrying ability of blood, and combined with an increase in heart rate produces an increase in blood pressure. This combination increases one's risk for a heart attack during or shortly following smoking marijuana. Even in experienced users, marijuana impairs a person's ability to remember events or information. Coordination, balance, and reaction time are also impaired.

RESPONSE TO ABRUPTLY STOPPING MARIJUANA

Addiction to marijuana does not seem to occur in all users; however, long-term marijuana use can lead to addiction. In those people who use marijuana compulsively, it will start to interfere with schoolwork, family life, and even recreational activities. People attempting to quit marijuana use report a variety of symptoms as follows.

1. Irritability
2. Restlessness

3. Nervousness
4. Decrease in appetite
5. Insomnia
6. Weight loss

Other side effects can include tremor, increased body temperature, an alteration in rapid eye movement (REM) sleep, and chills.

All of these symptoms are relatively mild compared to other drugs and they tend to only last for 4–5 days. However, in the long-term user, studies have demonstrated that marijuana can be a "gateway" drug to the use of other more addicting drugs (Lynsky et al., 2003).

An often overlooked health risk presented by marijuana use is that marijuana has the potential to produce lung cancer and other diseases of the respiratory tract. Marijuana smoke contains 50–70% more carcinogenic hydrocarbons than tobacco, information seldom reported by the anti-smoking movement. The style of smoking marijuana also contributes to the prolonged exposure to carcinogens, as marijuana smokers inhale more deeply and hold the smoke in their lungs longer.

SPICE DRUGS OR SYNTHETIC CANNABINOIDS

Synthetic cannabinoids were first detected in herbal mixtures in 2008 (Fattore and Fratta, 2011) and called "spice drugs" or "legal highs." While they did not contain cannabis, they did have the same or similar effect as THC, resulting in intoxication, psychosis, death, and withdrawal symptoms. These drugs are readily available over the internet and cannot be detected by conventional drug screening tests. The composition of the "spice drugs" is extremely variable, as is the potency. This variability lends itself to dangerous, and occasionally lethal outcomes.

MECHANISM OF ACTION

The mechanism of action of "spice," K2, KWH-018, to name a few, (collectively referred to as spice drugs) is similar to cannabis, only stronger. While THC is a partial agonist at the CB1 and CB2 receptors, the spice drugs act as full agonists (Atwood et al., 2010). Spice drugs have a higher affinity for both the CB1 and CB2 receptors than THC.

CENTRAL EFFECTS OF THE SPICE DRUGS

While there is not a lot of information on the effects of the spice drugs, Schifano and coworkers (2009) described the effects as "energizing, euphoric and disinhibiting." These effects are similar to those most sought after by marijuana users. Other less desirable effects that have been reported after chronic use are cognitive impairment, loss of consciousness, confusion, seizures, and unresponsiveness (Zimmerman et al., 2009.; Seely et al., 2011). Extreme anxiety accompanied by a sudden and severe depression has also been reported during withdrawal (Zimmerman et al., 2009.).

The spice drugs, thus far identified, contain synthetic cannabinoids that act as full agonists at the CB1 receptor. This increases the potency of the drug and the duration of action, thereby increasing the likelihood of an adverse reaction or serious side effect. Several suicides, coronary ischemic events and extreme and unbearable anxiety have been reported (Gay, 2010).

PERIPHERAL EFFECTS

The peripheral effects can be divided into two different groups. The unpleasant side effects, such as nausea, vomiting, and retching are the most common complaints (Fattore and Fratta, 2011). The second group consists of the dangerous side effects, such as extremely elevated heart rate and blood pressure, chest pain, and cardiac ischemia which are far more serious (Seely et al., 2011; Simmons et al., 2011). Spice drugs were also shown to alter metabolism in some users producing hypokalemia, hyperglycemia acidosis hyperthermia, and mydriasis (Simmons et al., 2011).

The ingredients found in "spice drugs" are variable, and the effect on both the central and peripheral nervous system potentially severe. This combination has proven difficult for emergency room health-care providers, as it is impossible to assess and treat the drug-related medical and psychiatric effects derived from the use of these synthetic cannabinoids.

ROUTE OF ADMINISTRATION

The spice drugs are a mixture of a variety of herbs and other vegetable matter to which the synthetic cannabinoids are then sprayed or added in some way. This mixture is then smoked (Fattore and Fratta, 2011).

Due to the limited data on this group of synthetic cannabinoids, the wide variety of ingredients in the "spice drugs" and the potential for serious damage to the user, the risk hardly seems to warrant the "legal high" obtained by using the synthetic cannabinoids.

Review Questions

1. Discuss the cannabinoid receptor and the effects of THC on this receptor.
2. What are the central effects of the CB1 antagonist on behavior?
3. What is the percentage of carcinogens in a marijuana cigarette?
4. Why is there an increase in heart rate in the first time user of marijuana?
5. Does smoking marijuana alter short-term memory?
6. Is marijuana similar to other drugs that alter short-term memory?

REFERENCES AND ADDITIONAL READING

Andre VM, Cepeda C, Cummings DM, et al. 2010. Dopamine modulation of excitatory currents in the striatum is dictated by the expression of D1 or D2 receptors and modified by endocannabinoids. *Eur. J. Neurosci.* 31:14–28.

Atwood BK, Huffman J, Straiker A, Mackie K. 2010. JWH018, a common constituent of "spice" herbal blends, is a potent and efficacious cannabinoid CB1 receptor agonist. *Br. J. Pharmacol.* 160:133–140.

Bari M, Battista N, Pirazzi V, Maccarone M. 2011. The manifold actions of endocannabinoids on female and male reproductive events. *Front. Biosci.* 16:498–516.

DiNieri J, Wang X, Szutorisz H, et al. 2011. Maternal cannabis use alters ventral striatal dopamine D2 gene regulation in the offspring. *Biol. Psychiatry.* 70:763–769.

Fattore L, Fratta W. 2011. Beyond THC: The new generation of cannabinoid designer drugs. *Front. Behav. Neurosci.* 5:60–70.

Fehr KO, Kalant H (eds). 1983. *Cannabis and Health Hazards.* The Addiction Research Foundation, Toronto.

Fitzgerald MI, Shobin E, Pickel VM. 2012. Cannabinoid modulation of the dopaminergic circuitry: implications for limbic and striatal output. *Prog. Neuropsychopharmacol. Biol. Psychiatry.* 38(1):21–29.

Gay M. 2010. Synthetic marijuana spurs state bans. *New York Times*, July 10.

Grotenhermen F. 2003. Pharmacokinetics and pharmcodynamics of cannabinoids. *Clin. Pharmacokinet.* 42:327–360.

Hall WD, Lynskey M. 2005. Is Cannabis a Gateway Drug? Testing hypotheses about the relationship between Cannabis use and the use of other illicit drugs. *Drug Alcohol Rev.* 24:39–48.

Howlett AC, Bidaut-Russell M, Devane WA, Melvin LS, Johnson MR, Herkenham M. 1990. The cannabinoid receptor: biochemical, anatomical and behavioral characterization. *Trends Neurosci.* 13:420–423.

Iversen LL. 2008. *The Science of Marijuana*, 2nd edn. Oxford University Press, Oxford.

Jones RT. 1983. Cannabis and health. *Ann. Rev. Med.* 34:247–258.

Lynsky MT, Vink JM, Boomsma DI. 2003. Early onset cannabis use and progression to other drugs use. *Behav. Genet.* 36:195–200.

Mathias R. 1996. Marijuana impairs driving-related ability skills and workplace performance. NIDA notes Jan/Feb.

Moore THM, Zammit S, Lingford-Hughes A, et al. 2007. Cannabis use and risk of psychotic or affective mental health outcomes: a systematic review. *Lancet* 370:319–328.

National Survey on Drug Use and Health: National Results: Appendix G: Selected Prevalence Tables. US Department of Human Health and Services, 2007.

Onaivi ES, Leonard CM, Ishiguro H, et al. 2002. Endocannabinoids and cannabinoid receptor genetics. *Prog. Neurobiol.*66: 307–344.

Perez-Reyes M, Di Guiseppi S, Davis KH, Schindler VH, Cook DE. 1982. Comparison of effects of marihuana cigarettes of three different potencies. *Clin. Pharmacol. Ther.* 31:617–624.

Petersen DR. 1980. A longitudinal study of the effects of tobacco and cannabis exposure on lung function in young adults. *Addiction.* 20:1055–1061.

Pertersen RC (ed). 1980. Marijuana Research Findings: National Institute on Drug Abuse Research Monograph Series. US Government Printing Office. Washington, DC.

Results from the 2011 National Survey on Drug Use and Health. Available at http://www.samhsa.gov/data/NSDUH/2011SummNatFindDetTables/Index.aspx

Ricci G, Cacciola G, Altucci L, et al. 2007. Endocannabinoid control of sperm motility: the role of epididyus. *Gen. Comp. Endocrinol.* 153:320–322.

Rossato M, Pagano C, Vettor R. 2008. The cannabinoid system and male reproductive functions. *J. Neuroendocrinol.* 20(suppl. 1):90–93.

Schifano F, Corazza O, Deluca P, et al. 2009. Psychoactive drug or mystical incense? Overview of the online available information on spice products. *Int. J. Cult. Ment. Health.* 2:137–144.

Seely KA, Prather PL, James LP, Moran JH. 2011. Marijuana-based drugs: innovative therapeutics or designer drugs of abuse? *Mol. Interv.* 11:36–51.

Simmons J, Cookman L, Kang C, Skinner C. 2011. Three cases of "spice" exposure. *Clin. Toxicol.* 49:431–433.

Sofuoglu M, Sugarman DE, Carroll KM. 2010. Cognitive function as an emerging treatment target for marijuana addiction. *Exp. Clin. Psychopharmacol.* 18:109–119.

Substance Abuse and Mental Health Services Administration (SAMHSA). 2008. Office of Applied Studies: National Survey on Drug Use and Health. US Department of Health and Human Services, Washington, DC.

Substance Abuse and Mental Health Services Administration (SAMHSA). 2010. NSDUH: Latest National Survey on Drug Use and Health, Substance Abuse Data, SAMHSA, Office of Applied Studies. http://www.oas.samhsa/nsduhLatest.htm, accessed on January 23, 2011.

Svensson T. 2000. Dysfunctional brain dopamine systems induced by psychotomimetic NMDA-receptor antagonist and the effects of antipsychotic drugs. *Brain Res. Brain Res. Rev.* 31:320–329.

Topics in Brief: Marijuana. Available at http://www.drugabuse.gov/publicati ons/topics-in-brief/marijuana, accessed on January 15, 2013.

Wagner FA, Anthony JC. 2002. From first drug use to drug dependence; developmental periods of risk for dependence upon marijuana, cocaine, and alcohol. *Neuropsychopharmacology*. 26:479–488.

Wilson RI, Nicoll RA. 2002. Endocannabinoid signaling in the brain. *Science*. 296:678–682.

Zimmermann US, Winkelmann PR, Pilhatsch M, Nees JA, Spanagel R, Schulz K. 2009. Withdrawal phenomena and dependence syndrome after the consumption of "spice gold." *Dtsch. Artzebl. Int*. 106:464–467.

11 Inhalants and Miscellaneous Drugs

Learning Objectives

The student will learn:

1. What are the different categories of inhalants?
2. What are the central nervous system (CNS) effects of inhalants?
3. What is the mechanism of action of nitrites and organic nitrates?
4. The similarities between bath salts and cocaine and 3,4-methylene-dioxypyrovalerone (MDMA).
5. The central and peripheral effects of mephedrone.
6. The mechanism of action of Salvia.
7. The central and peripheral effects of Khat.
8. The long-term effects of these drugs.

A wide variety of drugs fall under the category of inhalants or volatile substances whose chemical vapors can be inhaled to produce a psychoactive effect (Figure 11.1). While there are other illegal drugs that are inhaled, the term "inhalant" is used to describe a drug that is not taken by any other route of administration. There are a variety of substances that can be found in the home or workplace that are volatile, and can be used to get high. While they are not commonly thought of as drugs, because they have another purpose, products such as glue, cleaning fluid, gasoline, paint thinner, or spray paints, all can produce intoxicating effects.

There are several categories of inhalants.

Volatile solvents: paint thinners, gasoline, degreasers, office supply solvents, felt-tip markers, and glue.

Aerosols: spray paints, hair sprays, fabric protector sprays, computer cleaning products, and vegetable oil sprays.

Drugs of Abuse: Pharmacology and Molecular Mechanisms, First Edition. Sherrel G. Howard.
© 2014 John Wiley & Sons, Inc. Published 2014 by John Wiley & Sons, Inc.

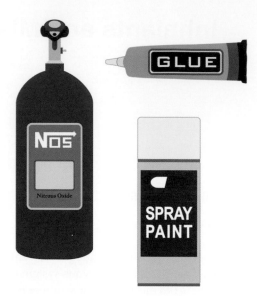

Figure 11.1   Inhalants

Gases: butane lighters, propane tanks, whipped cream aerosols or dispensers, refrigerant gases, and medical supplies such as ether, chloroform, halothane, and nitrous oxide (laughing gas).
Nitrites: organic nitrites are volatiles that include cyclohexyl, butyl, and amyl nitrites.

EFFECTS ON THE CENTRAL NERVOUS SYSTEM

The effects of inhalants on the central nervous system (CNS) can be mild, somewhat similar to alcohol. Using a small amount of inhalants can produce a lack of coordination, euphoria, dizziness, and slurred speech. With higher doses hallucinations or delusions can be experienced. As doses become larger, and the number of exposures increase the user can experience a loss of control, nausea, and vomiting. However, by displacing the air in the lungs, the body is deprived of oxygen. This is called hypoxia. Hypoxia results in damage to cells throughout the body, and the brain is particularly sensitive to a decrease in oxygen. The symptoms can vary depending on which area of the brain is most affected. Damage to the hippocampus will result in memory loss, so that a person with a damaged hippocampus will have difficulty learning or may have difficulty carrying on a normal conversation. Long-term use of inhalants can damage myelin, resulting in muscle spasms and tremors, or even difficulty walking and talking.

According to the National Institute of Drug Abuse (NIDA) reports in 2007, addiction to inhalants can occur with repeated abuse. While addiction is not a common occurrence, as the use of inhalants seems to be more popular with younger users. A mild withdrawal syndrome can occur with long-term use of inhalants. Studies have demonstrated that the use of inhalants does act as a "gateway" drug, when used at a younger age and can lead to further drug abuse throughout the adult years.

LETHAL EFFECTS

Abusers of inhalants risk a wide array of devastating medical consequences. The chemicals in solvents or aerosol sprays are highly concentrated and can induce irregular heart rhythms leading to fatal heart failure in minutes in a session of prolonged sniffing. This has been termed "sudden sniffing death" and usually results from sniffing butane, propane, or chemicals in aerosols. Inhalant abuse can also cause death according to NIDA reports (2007) by the following.

Asphyxiation: from displaced oxygen in the lungs.
Suffocation: from blocking the airways of the lungs when inhaling fumes from a plastic bag.
Seizures: from abnormal electrical discharges in the brain.
Coma: from the brain shutting down.
Choking: from inhalation of vomit after inhalant use.
Fatal injury: from car accidents occurring while intoxicated.

Both animal and human studies have demonstrated that most inhalants are extremely toxic. Not only are inhalants toxic to the brain, other organs are also damaged. Chronic exposure produces damage to the heart, lungs, liver, and kidneys. Some of this damage may be reversible; however, many syndromes caused by repeated and prolonged use of inhalants are not reversible.

AGE OF FIRST USE OF INHALANTS

Wu et al. (2005) determined that depending on the age of the adolescent starting to use inhalants there was a variation in the product chosen dependent on age.

Among new users: age 12–15. Inhalants used were glue, shoe polish, spray paints, gasoline, and lighter fluid.
Among new users: age 16–17. Inhalants used were nitrous oxide (laughing gas).
Among new users: adults. Inhalants used were nitrites.

Nitrites

Nitrite inhalants are still commonly abused in the United States. Historically, amyl nitrite was prescribed for angina pectoris, this was in the mid-1800s. Angina pectoris is the primary symptom in ischemic heart disease. It results in severe chest pain that radiates to the left shoulder and down the left arm. Angina pectoris can be induced by exercise, stress, or over eating. It was soon discovered that butyl nitrites also possessed the same vasodilatory qualities; however, butyl nitrite was not developed for clinical use. Sublingual tablets of nitroglycerin and later transdermal patches replaced amyl nitrite. However, amyl nitrite could still be purchased over-the-counter until 1960 when it was noticed, both by the FDA and manufacturers, that there was an increasing market for amyl nitrite by healthy males. The FDA reinstated the prescription requirement, initiating an underground market for amyl nitrite.

While amyl nitrite is still listed for angina pectoris, it is now primarily used by homosexual men or as an adjunct to other drugs (Chu et al., 2003). Scientific interest has increased in nitrites because of the possible link to AIDS and other sexually transmitted diseases.

MECHANISM OF ACTION

The nitrites and the organic nitrates dilate vascular and smooth muscles. This is accomplished by activating guanylate cyclase, thereby increasing the synthesis of cyclic GMP. Through a chain of events, leading to the formation of nitric oxide, and eventually to the dephosphorylation of myelin, and the relaxation of vascular and smooth muscles (Gilman et al., 1985).

NONMEDICAL NITRITE USE

The most commonly used inhalants in the United States are the alkyl nitrites (Haverkos et al., 1994). The use is varied according to gender, region of the country and race, with male high school seniors reporting the highest rates of inhalant use (Chu et al., 2003). Males are twice as likely to use inhalants as females (NIDA, 1993) and inhalant use was higher in the Northeast and lowest in the West. In adults, the use of nitrite inhalants has been predominantly associated with gay men and HIV transmission (Chu et al., 2003). It is also being considered as a cofactor in AIDS-related Kaposi's sarcoma.

BATH SALTS

Bath salts are "the newest kid on the block" of abused drugs. They are considered to be highly addictive psychoactive drugs that include

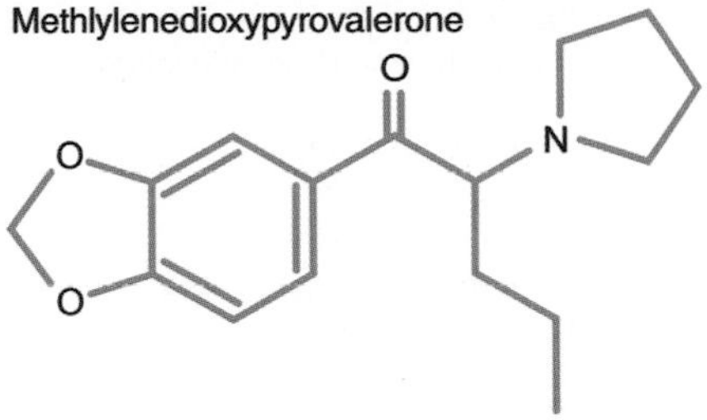

Methlylenedioxypyrovalerone

Figure 11.2 Structural formula for 3,4-methylene-dioxypyrovalerone (MDPV) "bath salts."

a variety of synthetic components, similar to cocaine and MDMA. The "high" that is produced from bath salts is comparable to the "high" from methamphetamine. The main ingredient in bath salts is 3,4-methylene-dioxypyrovalerone (MDPV), which is a psychoactive drug and classified as a Schedule V drug (Figure 11.2). MDPV was initially used as a research tool, and was a legal drug. However, it rapidly became abused as it was sold as an alternative to other drugs, such as cocaine. A second component of bath salts is mephedrone (4-methylmeth-cathinone). It is also a synthetic stimulant and contains cathinone. Mephedrone originally was derived from "khat," a plant that is grown primarily in Africa. When both compounds are present, it is called "herbal bath salts" since at least one component of the drug is plant derived.

Bath salts can also contain a variety of other compounds: 4-fluoromethcathinone, 3-fluorometh-cathinone, e-methoxymethcathinone, and 3,4 methylene-dioxymethcathinone (Methylone). This uncontrolled variety of compounds makes bath salts all the more dangerous for the consumer. There are a wide variety, which are sold under names such as blue silk, vanilla sky, route 69, and white rush. Herbal bath salts have a different, although no less interesting group of names, such as white dove, stardust, hurricane, cloud-9, etc. Bath salts are imported from India or China.

Route of Administration

Bath salts can be taken in any one of three ways: swallowed, inhaled, or injected. Snorting is the most common route of administration and injection is by far more dangerous. Snorting is the most common route of administration as the drug is sold in a "ready to snort" can, containing a 500 mg package of powder.

ADDICTION

Bath salts are addicting for the same reason that methamphetamine, MDMA, and cocaine are addicting. They produce a rapid euphoria and an increase in energy.

Table 11.1   Central and Peripheral Nervous System Effects of 3,4-methylene-dioxypyrovalerone

Increase heart rate	Hypertension
Vasoconstriction	Insomnia
Respiratory difficulty	Extreme excitement
Other Negative Symptoms	
Facial muscle tension	Nausea, stomach cramps
Tongue rolling	Pupil dilation
Bruxism	Kidney pain
Muscle fasciculation	Dizziness
Anxiety	Psychotic delusions
Panic attacks	Suicidal thoughts
Violent tendencies	Hallucinations

Bath salts produce effects similar to methamphetamine such as the following.

Initial rush or euphoria when injected.
They are an appetite suppressant.
They provide more energy.
Enhanced mental function.
Increased social behavior.
Increased libido.

There are a significant number of negative side effects that are also produced by bath salts. Among the most pronounced are found in Table 11.1.

The violent tendencies observed in bath salt abuse involved the user either committing suicide or violently murdering another person. In the cases of committing suicide in a violent manner, the user cut their own throat, face, or stomach. In the cases of violence against another person, the murders were particularly violent, beheadings, shootings, and stabbings. These episodes were probably due to hallucinations associated with high doses of bath salts. High doses of bath salts are probably very similar to high doses of amphetamines and/or cocaine. An average dose would be approximately 10 mg to produce the desired high. Since the bath salts are sold in 500 mg cans, the likelihood of an overdose would be very high.

Signs and Symptoms of Drug Overdose

The necessary research has not been done on the main ingredients of bath salts. It is possible to predict that bath salts will produce certain behaviors based on the structure of the primary compound in bath salts; however, a critical evaluation of this drug has not been made.

Much of the information on MDPV can be found in one research publication (Coppola and Mondola, 2012).

Table 11.2   Typical Symptoms of Withdrawal

Depression	Fatigue
Lethargy	Headache
Decreased appetite	Hypotension
Bloodshot eyes	

Symptoms of drug overdose
Mild fever
Dysphoria
Hypothermia
Hallucinations
Violent actions

Drug overdose seems to be a result of attempting to "tweak" bath salts. Similar tweaking is seen in cases of methamphetamine abuse and occasionally from MDMA abuse. This consists of the user taking an initial dose, which produces the expected "rush." When this initial euphoric effect wears off, the desire to reproduce it leads to "tweaking." At this time the majority of bath salts would not have been metabolized and cleared from the body, so the continued use increases the concentration in the body, resulting in an overdose. Similar types of "runs" can last for several days, and are very dangerous.

WITHDRAWAL SYMPTOMS

After extended "binges," there is a significant withdrawal period that is similar to that seen with methamphetamine withdrawal (Table 11.2).

MDPV is metabolized by P450 in the liver, methylcatechol and pyrrolidine are produced and these in turn are glucuronated and excreted by the kidneys. Only a small fraction is excreted in the fecal matter (Strano-Rossi et al., 2010).

MEPHEDRONE

Mephedrone is yet another designer drug, in a long series of designer drugs, used to evade the laws on illegal drugs. See the structural formula in Figure 11.3. The street names for mephedrone are meph, drone, and MCAT. Mephedrone was first synthesized in 1929 and was "rediscovered" in 2003. Between the years 2004 and 2008, a similar drug was legal in Israel and sold under the name "hagigat." Mephedrone was first available on the internet, and was used as an ecstasy substitute. Europol first became aware of its use in 2008, and noted that it could be found in Denmark, Finland, and the United Kingdom. Mephedrone was quickly replacing cocaine and MDMA, as the purity of cocaine fell from 60% to 22%, and

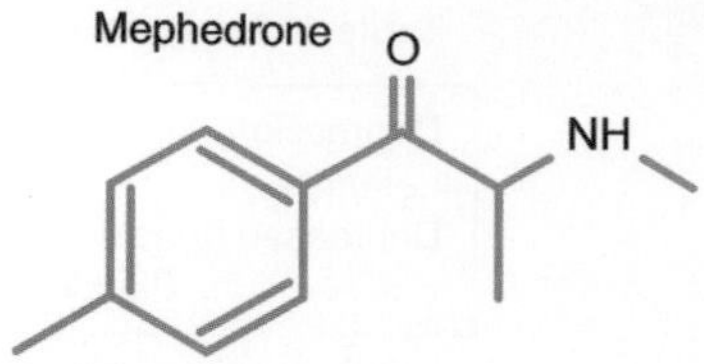

Figure 11.3   Structural formula for mephedrone.

MDMA pills seized in 2009 contained no MDMA. Similar patterns were observed throughout Europe.

There are few research studies on humans or animals that describe the effects of mephedrone. Therefore the description of the drug effects come from mephedrone users.

Reported effects of mephedrone include the following.
Euphoria, increased stimulation.
Elevated mood, decreased hostility.
Improved mental function.
Slight increase in sexual stimulation.

These effects would seem similar to those obtained from cocaine or amphetamine.

Routes of Administration

It is reported that when taken orally, the onset of action is approximately 15–30 minutes. When the drug is snorted, the effects occur almost immediately and peak within 30 minutes. Whether orally or nasally, the effects are over in 2–3 hours.

SIDE EFFECTS OF MEPHEDRONE

The following side effects were reported either by the European Monitoring Centre for Drugs and Drug Addiction (EMCDDA) or various hospitals within the United Kingdom. The side effects range from poor concentration, teeth grinding (bruxism), poor short-term memory, hallucinations, delusions, and erratic behavior. Other more serious side effects were generally the result of long-term use, or high-dose use of mephedrone, and consisted of increased body temperature, increased heart rate, breathing difficulties, anxiety, paranoia, and depression. There have been other reports of nausea, vasoconstriction, resulting in cold or blue extremities, headaches, seizures, and hypertension, usually coming from emergency room admissions.

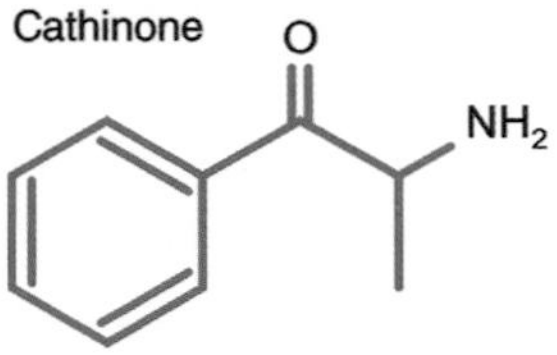

Cathinone

Figure 11.4   Structural formula for the active ingredient in khat, cathinone.

One study from the British Medical Journal (Winstock et al., 2010) stated that considering the chemical structure, mephedrone most likely stimulated release of catecholamines and inhibited the reuptake of norepinephrine (NE) and dopamine (DA). Since the cathinone derivatives act much like amphetamine, this would be a reasonable assumption. These authors concluded by saying that mephedrone appeared to be as harmful as ecstasy or amphetamine.

KHAT

Khat is a stimulant that is derived from a shrub in East Africa and southern Arabia. The use of Khat dates back thousands of years and is part of the social custom in these areas. Khat is pronounced "cot," and while the plant is not illegal, a chemical constituent of the plant, cathinone (Figure 11.4), is an illegal drug and has been listed as a Schedule I drug.

Khat contains an active ingredient cathinone, which is less potent than amphetamine, but is a psychoactive drug. Like amphetamine, it is a stimulant. The leaves of the plant are chewed producing a state of euphoria, increased arousal and alertness. Peripheral effects include an increase in heart rate and blood pressure, vasoconstriction, and the user may become more active and have a decreased appetite.

The effects of Khat generally last for 90 minutes to 3 hours, but have been reported to last longer. On withdrawal from Khat, the user is depressed, irritable, has difficulty sleeping, and may experience a loss of appetite.

LONG-TERM EFFECTS

Long-term use of Khat produces tooth decay and periodontal disease as well as constipation, ulcers, inflammation of the stomach and increased risk of cardiovascular problems. More serious long-term effects include depression, sometimes hallucinations, oral cancer and in some cases Khat precipitates psychosis.

TOLERANCE

It is not known if a tolerance or a physical dependence to Khat develops. Reports have cited nightmares and trembling on withdrawal that lasted for several days.

SALVIA

Salvia divinorum is a plant that is a native to Mexico. Salvia has been used by local healers and shamans as part of various rituals, and is known for its hallucinogenic properties. Salvia has become more popular because of its availability and ease of cultivation.

The active ingredient in Salvia is the diterpenoid, salvinorin A (Figure 11.5). It is present in the dried Salvia leaves in an amount of less than 0.2%. However, since it is active at a dose of ~200 mg, it is a particularly potent hallucinogen. Salvinorin A may in fact be the most potent, naturally occurring hallucinogen.

MECHANISM OF ACTION

Salvinorin A is a k-opioid receptor agonist (Roth et al., 2002) and it is also a very potent partial agonist at the DA D_2 receptor. It is not a "classic" hallucinogen, as it does not interact with the 5-HT$_{2A}$ receptor, as would be expected based on drugs like lysergic acid diethylamide (LSD) and mescaline. Salvinorin A has been used by shamans in Mexico and produces intense hallucinations lasting about 60 minutes (Cunningham et al., 2011).

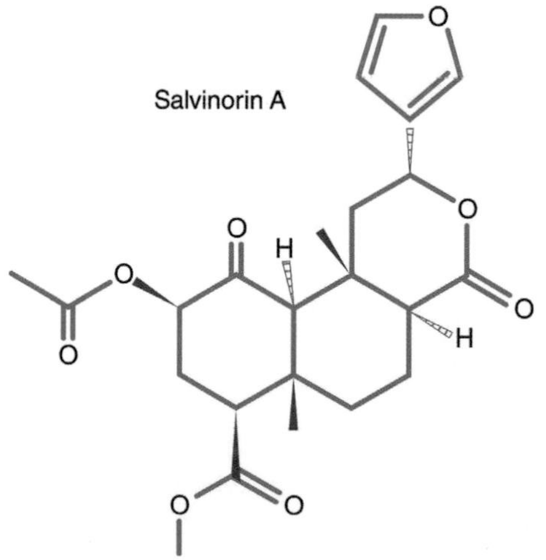

Salvinorin A

Figure 11.5   Structural formula for the active ingredient salvinorin A.

Medicinal Use

The leaves of the plant are used by traditional healers to treat ailments such as diarrhea, headaches, rheumatism, and is being tested for possible analgesic activity (Carlezon et al., 2005).

ROUTES OF ADMINISTRATION

Traditional methods used by healers or shamans consisted of crushing leaves to extract the juices. The juices or even some leaves were mixed to produce an infusion or tea, which was drunk in a healing ceremony.

Modern methods of ingestion consist of smoking or chewing the leaf. When Salvia is smoked, the effects occur very quickly, reaching a peak within 1 minute and lasting for approximately 5–10 minutes. The user returns to normal within 20 minutes with all effects of the drug gone.

When chewing the leaves, salvinorin A is absorbed through the oral mucosa. The leaves are not swallowed, but rather spit out. Salvinorin A is metabolized by the P450-mediated degradation that followed Michaelis–Menten kinetics (Cunningham et al., 2011).

EFFECTS OF SALVINORIN A

There has been very little research on the effects of Salvia in research animals or humans. Many of the reported effects are derived from a compilation of reported effects from users, and as such may have limited reliability. The reported effects can be divided into three groups as follows.

Short-term effects
Uncontrollable laughter
Merging with objects
Kinesthetic experiences
Trance-like state
A sense of motion

Intermediate effects that remain after initial peak effect are the following.

Increased insight	Decreased insight
Increased sweating	Decreased sweating
Feels warm	Feels cold
Increased confidence	Decreased confidence
Improved concentration	Difficulty concentrating

Other commonly reported feelings of: calmness, floating feelings, light-headed, and mind racing.

Long-term effects: The long-term effects of *Salvia divinorum* are equally at odds, and this probably reflects the lack of research on this subject. It is established that salvinorin A is a k-opioid agonist, and would be expected to produce dysphoria in humans. However, there are reports of it being used as a self-medication in the treatment of depression. Many respondents have reported an improved mood after using Salvia. Other respondents have reported long-lasting anxiety.

Extracts of Salvia have recently been developed, and the extracts are considerably more potent. The effects of this new and improved, more potent Salvia remains to be seen.

Review Questions

1. Discuss the lethal effects of the inhalants.
2. What are the results of the hypoxia produced by inhalants?
3. Discuss the positive and negative effects of bath salts.
4. Based on the chemical structure of mephedrone, the mechanism of action should most resemble which drugs?
5. Why would Salvia act as an analgesic?

REFERENCES AND ADDITIONAL READING

Carlezon WA, Beguin C, DiNieri JA, et al. 2005. Depressive-like effects of the k-Opioid receptor agonist salvinorin A on behavior and neurochemistry in rats. *J. Pharmacol. Exp. Ther.* 316:440–447.

Chu PL, McFarland W, Gibson S, et al. 2003. Viagra use in a community-recruited sample of men who have sex with men, San Francisco. *J. Acquir. Immune Defic. Syndr.* 33:191–193.

Coppola M, Mondola R. 2012. 3,4-Methylene-dioxypyrovalerone (MDPV): Chemistry, pharmacology and toxicology of a new designer drug of abuse marketed online. *Toxicol. Letters.* 208:12–15.

Cunningham CW, Rothman RB, Prisinzano TE. 2011. Neuropharmacology of the naturally occurring κ-opioid hallucinogen salvinorin A. *Pharmacol. Rev.* 63:316–347.

Europol-EMCDDA. 2010. Joint report on a new psychoactive substance: 4-methylmethcathinone (mephedrone). European Monitoring Center for Drugs and Drug Addiction.

Giannini AJ, Castellani S. 1982. A manic-like psychosis due to khat. *J. Toxicol. Clin. Toxicol.* 19:455–459.

Gilman AG, Goodman SD, Rall TW, Murad F. 1985. *Goodman and Gilman's The Pharmacological Basis of Therapeutics.* Macmillan, New York.

Haverkos HW, Drotman DP, Morgan WM. 1994. Kaposi's sarcoma in patients with AIDS: sex, transmission mode and race. *Biomed. Pharmacother*. 44:461–466.

Institute for Social Research. Monitoring the Future. 2009. Study Results. Ann Arbor, MI. University of Michigan. http://www.monitoringthefuture.org

National Institute on Drug Abuse (NIDA). 1993. Smoking, drinking and illicit drug use among American secondary school students, college students, and young adults, 1975–1991. Volume 1. *Secondary Students*. NIH Publication no. 93-3400, Rockville, MD.

National Institute on Drug Abuse (NIDA) Reports. 2007. Inhalant Abuse. Bethesda, MD.

Romanelli F, Smith KM, Thornton AC, Pomeroy C. 2004. Poppers: epidemiology and clinical management of inhaled nitrite abuse. *Pharmacotherapy*. 24:69–78.

Roth B, Baner K, Westkaemper R, et al. 2002. Salvinorin A: a potent naturally occurring non-nitrogenous kappa k opioid selective agonist. *Proc. Natl. Acad. Sci USA*. 99:11934–11939.

Strano-Rossi S, Cadwallader A, De La Torre X, Botre F. 2010. Toxicological determination and in vitro metabolism of the designer drug methylenedioxypyrovalerone(MDPV) by gas chromatography/mass spectrometry and liquid chromatography/quadrupole time of flight mass spectrometry. *Rapid Commun. Mass Spectrom*. 24:2706–2714.

Substance Abuse and Mental Health Services Administration. 2008. The NSDUH Report: Inhalant Use across the Adolescent Years. April 2008.

Turner DM. 1996. *Effects and Experiences: Salvinorin-The Psychedelic Essence of Salvia Divinorum*. Panther Press, San Francisco, CA.

Winstock A, Marsden J, Metcheson L. 2010. What should be done about mephedrone? *British Med. J*. 340:c1605.

Wu LT, Schlenger WE, Ringwalt CL. 2005. Use of nitrite inhalants ("poppers") among American youth. *J. Adolesc. Health*. 37:52–60.

Part VI   Recovery and Relapse

12 Treatment of Substance Dependency

Mark DeAntonio

The risk of any drug use is drug abuse and drug addiction or dependence. DSM IV states "The essential feature of dependence is a cluster of cognitive, behavioral, and physiological symptoms indicating that the individual continues substance use despite significant substance related problems." Any substance use can lead to either physiological or behavioral dependence and often both.

According to the Substance Abuse and Mental Health Services Administration's (SAMHSA's) National Survey on Drug Use and Health, 23.5 million persons aged 12 or older needed treatment for an illicit drug or alcohol abuse problem in 2009 (9.3% of persons aged 12 or older). Of these, only 2.6 million—11.2% of those who needed treatment—received it at a specialty facility.

The path to drug dependency has multiple factors. These functions have different weights over the course of substance dependency. Initially substance availability, social acceptability, and peer modeling lead to experimentation and use. The level of cognitive function and personality traits can reinforce chronic use, which in turn modifies neurophysiologic functions, thus reinforcing dependency. Social and economic factors also have influence as well as environmental (i.e., traumatic) and psychiatric illnesses. Additionally, specific substances have different degrees of central nervous system influence that more or less intensifies the experience and promotes dependence. There are further complications due to individual responses to substances at a neurophysiologic level that allow an individual to be more or less vulnerable to dependency. These factors are familial or genetic, and are independent of environment or parenting. Finally there is clear evidence that the age of onset of substance use is a strong factor or determinator in dependency formation. Individuals initiating substance use in late childhood or early adolescence have significantly higher rates of substance dependency.

Drugs of Abuse: Pharmacology and Molecular Mechanisms, First Edition. Sherrel G. Howard.
© 2014 John Wiley & Sons, Inc. Published 2014 by John Wiley & Sons, Inc.

Not everyone who uses a substance becomes dependent. In the United States, a majority of young adults in college experiment with substance use. However many, upon graduation, do not continue substance use and do not develop a dependence. However, continual substance use over 3–6 months, regardless of the substance used, results in changes in neurologic functions that predict dependence. When substance dependence develops, it disrupts an individual's life at many levels. One's career, interpersonal functioning, family functioning, health, and functioning in the community are significantly affected. Intervention and treatment therefore is multidimensional and often not straightforward. There is rarely a "quick fix" and treatment is usually a long-term proposition, lasting years if not a lifetime.

The National Institute on Drug Abuse has published the following principles on effective treatment.

1. Addiction is a complex but treatable disease that affects brain function and behavior.
2. No single treatment is appropriate for everyone.
3. Treatment needs to be readily available.
4. Effective treatment attends to multiple needs of the individual, not just his or her drug abuse.
5. Remaining in treatment for an adequate period of time is critical.
6. Counseling, individual, and/or group, and other behavioral therapies are the most commonly used forms of drug abuse treatment.
7. Medications are an important element of treatment for many patients, especially when combined with counseling and other behavioral therapies.
8. An individual's treatment and services plan must be assessed continually and modified, as necessary to ensure that it meets his or her changing needs.
9. Many drug-addicted individuals also have other mental disorders.
10. Medically assisted detoxification is only the first stage of addiction treatment and by itself does little to change long-term drug abuse.
11. Treatment does not need to be voluntary to be effective.
12. Drug use during treatment must be monitored continuously, as lapses during treatment do occur.
13. Treatment programs should assess patients for the presence of HIV/AIDS, hepatitis B and C, tuberculosis, and other infectious diseases, as well as provide targeted risk-reduction counseling to help patients modify or change behaviors that place them at risk of contracting or spreading infectious diseases.

When substance dependence develops it becomes a chronic disorder. There can be periods of non-use, but relapses into dependence are expected. Because of this chronicity, treatment is a long-term commitment and rarely is short-term treatment effective.

There is no one treatment for substance dependence and while some substances, like opiates may have unique interventions, most treatments apply to all substance dependencies.

The most effective treatment programs provide a combination of therapies to meet the need of an individual's dependency issues.

Since the consequences of substance dependency's can be individual and complex, different treatment settings need to be employed to address a person's needs. Inpatient residential, partial hospital, insensitive outpatient, and outpatient settings can also be employed, reflecting the substance and severity of the dependency. Within each setting a multimodal treatment approach is applied. Individual, groups, couples, and family interventions should be available and considered. The need for lesser levels of restrictive treatment (inpatient being most restrictive, individual outpatient or group outpatient being least restrictive) needs to be regularly evaluated.

The first treatment intervention is often a detoxification program. This is a process where the individual is "detoxified" from the substance of dependency by stopping use. Stopping use results in withdrawal effects which may be physiologic and can be life threatening to severe anxiety, agitation, and substance cravings. A physician in an inpatient, residential, or outpatient setting with medications to address withdrawal symptoms manages the withdrawal. Historically detoxification was with medications similar in pharmacologic effect to the substance of dependence, using a less euphoric opiate to treat heroin withdrawal. Most detoxification programs use pharmacologic interventions that are not "legal" analogs of substances of abuse, though they can still control withdrawal symptoms. The detoxification of stimulants and cocaine often requires the use of antianxiety agents and antipsychotic agents to address withdrawal symptoms of agitation, paranoia, confusion, and extreme anxiety. After detoxification, which may last days to weeks, there needs to be a re-evaluation of the individual, to determine what the appropriate next level of treatment will be. Detoxification on its own never fully addresses substance dependency and if no further treatment is done, relapse would be expected.

The most restrictive level of treatment is residential treatment. Long-term residential treatment provides a treatment environment for 6–12 months. It is a highly structured, comprehensive program that through individual, group and social interventions, a patient is resocialized to change patterns of interacting and problem solving that lead to substance use and dependency. The intensive treatment allows someone to function, be productive, and interact socially without the need for using substances. Employment and educational services can be part of the treatment. This treatment is often employed with substance-dependent individuals who are part of the criminal justice system. There is also short-term residential treatment lasting 3–6 weeks. This is for individuals who do not require the resocialization interventions of long-term treatment, but require an intensive therapeutic intervention, using individual and group modalities, which can then continue in an outpatient setting for 6–12 months.

Outpatient treatment programs vary from 5 days a week, all-day partial hospital programs, to 3 days a week, 2–4 hours a day intensive outpatient programs to multiple days a week individual and group therapy programs. These programs allow individuals to continue in occupational settings and continue to maintain social supports if those supports are not involved in substance use. While less intense, these programs need to last 12 months or longer to be effective.

Pharmacologic interventions for treatment have been shown to be efficacious for opioid addiction. Three interventions have been shown to have efficacy: methadone, buprenorphine, and naltrexone. Methadone is a long-acting opioid, which is taken orally and produces little if any euphoria. However, due to its addictive potential and fatal overdose potential it is federally mandated to be dispensed in specialized outpatient treatment settings. It is effective in preventing opioid withdrawal, and additionally blocking the effects of simultaneous nonmethadone opiate use. It has drawbacks of often causing depression and insomnia.

Buprenorphine can also be used. It is a partial agonist and carries a low risk of overdose. Administration controls opioid withdrawal symptoms. There is no requirement for buprenorphine to be dispensed in specialty clinics, so treatment can be dispensed in outpatient offices, increasing access, and flexibly of treatment as individuals can take the medication at home and not in a clinic setting. This allows individuals to continue their regular occupational and social activities. Naltrexone is an orally administered opioid antagonist that is effective up to 72 hours after one administration. Because it is such an effective opioid antagonist, an individual will feel no effect of self-administered opioids. Naltrexone itself is not psychoactive or addictive. Therefore, it needs no unique medical supervision. However an individual needs to be highly motivated for compliance.

These three psychopharmacologic interventions—methadone, buprenorphine, and naltrexone—are only effective treatments when combined with behavioral and social interventions to motivate continued compliance and overall treatment. Other pharmacologic interventions have been proposed, focusing mostly on amphetamines and cocaine, but have not been shown to be efficacious. There are pharmacologic interventions for ethanol and nicotine, but those are not covered in this chapter.

Behavioral therapies are the primary interventions for successful substance abuse treatment. While first employed for alcohol abuse in the 1800s, they have been successfully modified to address non-alcohol substance dependency since the late 1900s. Behavioral therapies engage individuals in strategies that promote long-term change in behavior, problem solving, peer relationship, and goal-directed pursuits. Their goal is to promote psychological, interpersonal, and social competency, free of substance dependency. A number of behavioral interventions have been employed and shown validation in research studies. Cognitive behavioral therapy, matrix model, and 12-step facilitation therapy have the widest applicability and efficacy.

Cognitive behavioral therapy has been shown to be effective in treating a number of psychiatric disorders including depression, obsessive–compulsive disorder, and anxiety disorders. Research has documented its utility in preventing relapse for marijuana, cocaine, and methamphetamine dependency. The focus of treatment is to first identify behaviors that promote substance use. Cognitive strategies are employed to learn new behaviors that promote abstinence. Cognitive strategies are also developed to promote self-control of impulses that lead to dependence. The goal is to understand environmental and emotional triggers of substance use so an individual can have a proactive strategy to address these triggers. Articulating coping strategies that maintain sobriety are reinforced.

The Matrix Model has been shown to be effective for treatment of amphetamine and cocaine-dependent individuals. This treatment employs a variety of strategies to promote engagement in treatment and abstinence. There are psychoeducational, cognitive, supportive, 12-step groups and urine testing interventions coordinated by a therapist. Interventions are manualized and additionally include family and multifamily interventions.

12-Step Facilitation Therapy has been shown to be effective in treating opiate, cocaine, and amphetamine dependence. The intervention is engagement in 12-step self-help groups. Groups, especially in the first 3 months are attended at least daily. The focus of the groups is on the chronic illness model of substance dependence that is out of the control of the individual. Abstinence is essential, but cannot be found through will power, but by giving oneself over to a higher power, with the support of the other substance-dependent individuals in the group. The group focuses on social activities and interactions that maintain abstinence. While shown to be most effective with alcohol dependence, there is research showing efficacy over the long term with opiates, cocaine, and amphetamines. 12-step facilitation therapy can also be incorporated with other behavioral treatment modalities.

It is often asked if substance dependency treatment really works. Relapse is erroneously seen as failure. However, if one sees substance dependency as a chronic illness, then relapse is an expected occurrence. Hypertension, diabetes, asthma all have relapses. Instead of seeing recurrence of the illness as a failure, it needs to be seen as an opportunity to re-evaluate the treatment. One needs to analyze what factors caused the relapse and address them. This makes treatment a dynamic process adjusting the multitudes of interventions to meet the evolving needs of the dependent person.

REFERENCES AND ADDITIONAL READING

Strain A. 2009. Substance-related disorders. In: Comprehensive Textbook of Psychiatry. 9th edn. pp 1237–1431. [ED's: BJ Sadock, VA Sadock and P Ruiz.] Lippincot, Williams and Wilkins, Philadelphia, PA.

Diagnostic and Statistical Manual of Mental Disorder (DSM). 1994. *Substance-Related Disorders*, 4th edn. pp 175–272.

National Institute on Drug Abuse (NIDA). 2011. *Drug Facts: Treatment Statistics*. Revised March 2011.

National Institute on Drug Abuse (NIDA). 2009. *Principles of Drug Addiction Treatment: A Research Based Guide*. Revised April 2009.

Index

A

a-amino-3-hydroxy-5-methylisoxazole-4-
    propionic acid (AMPA), 29–30,
    30*f*
Ambion, 78
amphetamine. *See also* methamphetamine;
    methylenedioxymethamphetamine
  abuse of, 42
  animal studies, 38
  animal studies, mechanism of action, 40
  blocking the effect of, 39–40
  causes of death related to, 43
  central effect, 37
  conditioned response studies, 38–39
  dopamine (DA), d-amphetamine
    structures, 34*f*
  dopamine (DA), glutamate interactions
    and, 43, 44*f*
  dopamine (DA) system effect, 36
  first synthesis, 5, 33
  5-HT transporter (SERT) interaction,
    35–36
  human studies, 38
  indirectly acting sympathomimetics, 34
  mechanism of action, 34–36, 35*f*
  monoamine oxidase (MAO) and, 34
  Parkinson's patients, L-DOPA and, 39
  peripheral effect, 38
  pharmacokinetics, 44
  psychomotor stimulant, 36–37
  psychosis, 42–43
  stereotypical behavior development and,
    39
  student popularity, 38
  tolerance, dependence, 43
  transporter models, 35, 35*f*
  weight loss and, 5
amphetamine, clinical use
  appetite suppressant, 40–41
  attention deficit hyperactivity disorder
    (ADHD), 41

depression, 46
  narcolepsy treatment, 41
anxiolytic drugs, classes, 81*t*

B

barbiturates. *See also* benzodiazepines
  acute poisoning, treatment, 87–88
  addiction treatment, 88
  cardiovascular, respiratory systems
    effect, 90–91
  chronic use, events timeline, 86
  CNS distribution, 89, 89*t*
  GABA$_A$ receptor, 86–87
  general structure, 78*f*
  mechanism of action, 86
  pharmacodynamics of sedation and,
    89–90
  physical dependence in elderly, 88–89
  pregnant or nursing female use, 89
  site of action, 89*t*
  tolerance, dependence, 85–86
bath salts
  3,4 methylene-dioxypyrovalerone
    (MDPV) structure, 171, 171*f*
  addiction to, 170–172
  CNS, peripheral nervous system effects,
    171
  drug overdose signs, symptoms, 172–173
  route of administration, 171
  withdrawal symptoms, 173*t*
behavioral therapies, 186–187
benzodiazepines
  absorption rate, 84
  cardiovascular, respiratory systems
    effect, 90–91
  categories, 76
  Clinical uses, 90
  CNS distribution, 89, 89*t*
  dose–response curve and, 78, 79*f*
  γ-aminobutyric (GABA) and, 79–80, 80*f*
  half-life, 84–85, 85*t*

Drugs of Abuse: Pharmacology and Molecular Mechanisms, First Edition. Sherrel G. Howard.
© 2014 John Wiley & Sons, Inc. Published 2014 by John Wiley & Sons, Inc.

benzodiazepines (*Continued*)
  interaction at regulatory site, 87*f*
  mechanism of action, 79–81
  paradoxical effect, 81
  pharmacodynamics of sedation and,
    89–90
  pharmacokinetics, 84–85
  pharmacological effects, 81*t*
  physical dependence, 81, 81*t*
  physical dependence in elderly, 88–89
  pregnant or nursing female use, 89
  sedative hypnotic, 77–78
  site of action, 89*t*
  tolerance, dependence, 85–86
  toxicity, 85
  withdrawal from, 81–84
benzodiazepines, withdrawal symptoms
  conditions altering duration, intensity, 82
  elimination, factors influencing, 83–84
  exposure duration and, 82–83
  long-term outcomes, 83–84
  withdrawal response, factors
    influencing, 83
benzoylecgonine (BE), methylecgonine
    ester (MEE) metabolites, 69–70
Biosynthesis of DA and NE, 16–18

C
caffeine, nicotine, alcohol, 8
cocaine, 66–667, 67*f*
  benzoylecgonine (BE) and
    methlecgonine ester (MEE)
    metabolites, 69–70
  chronic use, toxic effects, 68
  CNS effects, 67
  crack cocaine, 69
  dopamine transporter (DAT) protein
    blockade, 66–66, 67*f*
  effects *vs.* methamphetamine, 48*t*
  historical use, 5, 65
  mechanism of action, 66–67, 67*f*
  metabolism, 69–70
  peripheral nervous system effects, 68
  pharmacokinetics, 69
  physical dependence, withdrawal, 68–69
  serotonin (5-HT) and, 66
  structural formula, 56*f*
  tolerance, 69–70
cocaine, neurobiology of relapse
  cocaine use, seeking, 70
  cross reinstatement and, 72
  dopamine (DA) receptors and, 71

  drug priming, 70–71
  glutamate and reinstatement, 72–73
  mesocorticolimbic DA system and, 71
  neurotransmitters involved, 71
  reinstatement models, 70–73
  stress-induced reinstatement, 71
codeine, 128
cognitive behavioral therapy, 187
combination therapies, 185
CNS stimulants, categories, 37
Cross-tolerance, 72

D
Dale, Sir Henry, 15
delta-9-tetrahydrocannabinol (THC). *See*
    marijuana
dependence, 9–10
dependence-producing drugs, common
    attributes, 10–11
detoxification programs, 185
dihydroxyphenylalanine (DOPA)
    decarboxylase, 17–18, 17*f*
dopamine (DA)
  biosynthesis of, 16–18, 17*f*
  cocaine, neurobiology of relapse, 71
  DA transporter (DAT), 20
  depletion,
    methylenedioxymethamphetamine
    (MDMA), 57
  drug-receptor interaction and, 20, 21*f*
  GHB and, 107–108
  glutamic acid (GLU) interaction, 31, 31*f*,
    43, 44*f*
  impulse flow, γ hydroxybutyrate (GHB),
    107–108
  metabolism, 19*f*, 20
  receptor subtypes, 21–22, 22*t*
  receptors activation, 8
  release, regulation of release, 19–20, 19*f*
  storage, 19*f*, 20
  synthesis regulation, 18–19
  system effect, amphetamine, 36
  Uptake I, 19
dopamine transporter (DAT) protein, 20
  cocaine abuse and, 66–66, 67*f*
dopamine-β-hydroxylase (DBH), 18
drug addiction, defined, 9
drug, substance abuse. *See also* substance
    dependency, treatment
  defined, 9, 183
  dependence-producing drugs, common
    attributes, 10–11

history, unauthorized use, 1–2
reward pathways, 10
reward pathways and, 10
society's attitude towards, 8
drug-receptor interaction, 20, 21*f*

E
ergot, 5–6, 6*f*, 138. *See also* LSD, 138
excitatory amino acid receptors. *See also*
    glutamic acid
    a-amino-3-hydroxy-5-methylisoxazole-4-
        propionic acid (AMPA), 29–30,
        30*f*
    kainic acid (KA), 30, 30*f*
    N-methyl-D-aspartate (NMDA), 29–31,
        30*f*, 31*f*
    subtypes, 29–30

F
Falck–Hillarp fluorescent histochemical
    method, 16
flashbacks, 144

G
γ-aminobutyric acid (GABA), 26
    benzodiazepines and, 79–80, 80*f*
    GABA_A receptor, 28, 28*f*, 80
    GABA_B receptor, 28–29, 80
    GHB and, 107
    released, 27, 27*f*
    storage, 27
    structure, 80*f*
    synthesis, 27
γ hydroxybutyrate (GHB)
    abuse potential, 111
    alcohol withdrawal, heroin addiction
        treatment, 109–110
    chemical structure, 106*f*
    dopamine (DA), impulse flow and,
        107–108
    effects on CNS, 106–107
    GABA receptors and, 107
    mechanisms of action, 105–107
    overdose symptoms, 111
    pharmacokinetics, 111
    synthesis, metabolism, 105–106, 106*f*
    therapeutic uses, narcolepsy treatment,
        108–109
glutamic acid (GLU), 29
    dopamine (DA) interaction, 31, 31*f*
    glutamine synapse, 30*f*
    synthesis, 29

H
Halcion, 75
hallucinogens. *See also* lysergic acid
        diethylamide; mescaline
    classes of, 142
    ergot, 5–6, 6*f*, 138
    hallucination, defined, 139
    hallucination persisting perception
        disorder (HPPD), 143–144
    historical use, 5–6, 137
    symptoms, 137–138
hemp, 7, 153. *See also* marijuana
heroin. *See* opium, morphine, heroin
Hoffmann, Albert
    synthesis of LSD, 6, 137-139
5-HT. *See* serotonin
5-hydroxytryptamine, *See* Serotonin, 22–26

I
inhalants
    addiction to, 168–169
    age of first use of, 169
    effects on CNS, 168–169
    lethal effects, 169
    mechanism of action, 170
    nitrites, 170
    nonmedical nitrite use, 170
    types, categories, 167–168, 168*f*

K
kainic acid (KA), 30, 30*f*
Khat
    active ingredient, 175
    historical use, 175
    long-term effects, 175
    structural formula, 175*f*
    tolerance, physical dependence to, 176

L
librium, 77
lysergic acid diethylamide (LSD)
    behavioral models, mechanism of action,
        140
    candy flipping, MDMA, 146–147, 146*t*,
        147*f*
    CNS effects of, 142–143
    flashbacks, hallucination persisting
        perception disorder (HPPD), 143–144
    hallucinogenic effects of, 58–59
    5-HT receptor neurons, 140–141, 141*f*
    long-term effects of, 143–144
    mechanism of action, 139–141, 141*f*

lysergic acid diethylamide (LSD)
   (*Continued*)
   mood alterations and, 143
   Passie Hypothesis and, 140–141
   peripheral nervous system effects of, 142,
     142*t*
   pharmacokinetics, 145
   physiological side effects of, 142, 142*t*
   psychosis, 143
   routes of administration, 144–145
   structure, 138*f*
   synesthesia and, 143
   synthesis, 6, 138–139
   toxicity, tolerance, 144–145

M
marijuana
   antimotivational syndrome, 158–159
   cannabinoid receptors CB1, CB2, 155–156
   CB1 receptor antagonist, CNS effects, 158
   CB1 receptors, neuroanatomical
     distribution, 156
   chronic, long-term use effects, 158, 159*t*,
     161
   endocrine changes, 159
   historical use, 6–7, 153–154
   leaf, 7*f*
   medicinal uses, 6–7
   response to abruptly stopping, 160–161
   synthesis, biosynthetic pathway, 154–155
   THC, clinical uses, 157–158
   THC, mechanism of action, 155–156
   THC, peripheral and CNS effects,
     156–157, 157*t*
   THC route of administration, absorption,
     159–160
   THC, structural formula, 154–155, 155*f*
   tolerance, addiction, physical
     dependence, 160
   U.S. consumption, 154
Matrix Model, 187
mephedrone (MCAT)
   effects, 174
   routes of administration, 174
   side effects, 174–175
   structural formula, 173, 174*f*
mescaline (peyote)
   central, peripheral nervous system
     effects, 148–149
   mechanism of action, 148
   pharmacokinetics, 149
   structural formula, 148*f*

mesocorticolimbic dopamine (DA) system
   cocaine, neurobiology of relapse, 71
methamphetamine
   abuse, 47, 48*t*
   adrenergic action, 46
   central, peripheral effects, 45
   clinical study, Japan, 47–49
   clinical uses, 45–46
   common, trade names, 45
   depression and, 46
   effects *vs.* cocaine, 48*t*
   metabolism, 50
   Parkinson's disease and, 46
   potential therapeutic uses, 47
   short-term effect, 49
   structure of, 44, 44*f*
   tolerance, dependence, 49–50
methylecgonineester (MEE), 69–70
3,4 methylene-dioxypyrovalerone (MDPV)
   structure, 171, 171*f*
methylenedioxymethamphetamine
   (MDMA)
   acute effects, 56
   acute withdrawal effects, 52*t*
   adolescent abuse, ecstasy, 50–51
   aggregation toxicity and, 57–58
   candy flipping, LSD, 146–147, 146*t*,
     147*f*
   clinical use, 50
   CNS effects, 51–52, 52*t*
   dopamine (DA) release, depletion and,
     57
   first synthesis, 50
   hallucinogenic effects of, 58–59
   mechnism of action, 51
   neuropsychiatric effects, cognitive
     impairment and, 52
   neurotoxicity, 52–53
   pharmacokinetics in humans, 60
   reinstatement of drug-seeking behavior
     and, 59–60
   serotonin (5-HT) effects of, 54–56, 54*f*
   serotonin (5-HT) syndrome, 58
   short- *vs.* long-term effects, 53*f*
   structural formula, 50*f*
   tryptophan hydroxylase inhibition by,
     56–57
monoamine oxidase (MAO)
   amphetamine and, 34
morphine. *See* opium, morphine, heroin
Mrs. Winslow's Soothing Syrup, 4, 119,
   120*t*

N

National Institute on Drug Abuse, effective treatment principles, 184

National Survey on Drug Use and Health (2003), 4

neurotransmission, biochemistry
    adrenergic transmission, 15
    historical overview, 15–16
    norepinephrine (NE), 15–16

Nitrites
    amyl nitrite, 170
    mechanism of action, 170
    non-medical use, 170

N-methyl-D-aspartate (NMDA) receptors, 29–31, 30f, 31f

norepinephrine (NE), 15–16. *See also* dopamine (DA)
    biosynthesis of, 16–17, 17f

O

opium. *See also* morphine, heroin
    addiction to opiates, 117–118
    affluent drug users, 4
    antagonists, 130
    central neurons effects, 126
    CNS effects, 123 124
    codeine, 128
    cognitive behavior-based treatment models, 132
    common use of, 4
    economics, Opium Wars, 3
    endogenous morphine, 124–126
    endorphin precursor molecules, 125–126
    G-protein coupled receptors (GPCRs), 121, 122f, 126–127
    heroin addiction, 127
    heroin consumption effects, 127
    heroin synthesis, 127
    history, 2–4, 118–120
    hypodermic needle invention, use, 3, 119
    immunotherapy and, 131–132
    mechanism of action, 4, 120–121, 121t
    morphine antagonists, naloxone, 130, 130t
    morphine naltrexone, 130–131, 130t
    nineteenth century use, 4
    opioid receptors, 121–122, 121t, 122f, 122t, 126
    opioid receptor distribution, 122, 122t
    opioid receptors, associated functional effects, 122, 123t
    opioid tolerance, 129

μ-opioid receptors, 121–123, 122t, 126
oxycodone, 128
OxyContin, 128–129
pain management and, 117, 132
pharmacokinetics, 129
physical dependence, withdrawal syndrome, 129–132
prescription drugs, 127–129
receptor subtypes interaction, 121t
seventeenth century opium, 3, 118, 120
Soldier's Disease, 3, 119
structural formula, 118
sympathetic nervous system effects, 124
thebaine (paramorphine), 128
tolerance and withdrawal, 129
treatment, 131–132
twentieth century use, 4, 120
Vietnam War addicts and, 4
Winslow's Soothing Syrup, 4, 119, 120f
Opium Wars, 3
outpatient treatment, 186
oxycodone, 128
OxyContin, 128–129

P

peyote. *See* mescaline
pharmacologic interventions, 186
phencyclidine (PCP), ketamine
    addiction, illicit use, 101–102
    advantages, side effects, 96
    clinical uses, 98, 100–101
    CNS effects, 97, 98t
    distribution, elimination, 102
    duration of action, 102–103
    effect on performance, 101–102
    effects at different dosages, 97, 98t
    gluatamate hypothesis of schizophrenia and, 99–100, 99t
    illicit use, 95–96
    mechanism of action, 96
    metabolism, 102
    neuropharmacology, 97–98, 98t
    NMDA receptor and, 96
    open channel blockers, 96
    peripheral nervous system effects, 97, 98t
    pharmacokinetics, 102–103
    routes of administration, 100
    schizophrenic patient, PCP user, 100
    structural formula, 97f
    withdrawal, 101
phenylethanolamine-N-methyltransferase, 18

physical withdrawal syndrome, 9
pleasure-seeking effect, 8
positive reinforcement, defined, 9
psychological dependence, defined, 9
Pure Food and Drug Act, 4, 119

R
residential treatment, 185–186

S
salvia *(salvia divinorum)*
  medicinal use, 177
  routes of administration, 177
  salvinorin A, effects, 177–178
  salvinorin A, structural formula, 176*f*
  traditional use, 176
serotonin (5-HT)
  biosynthesis of, 22–23, 23*f*, 24*f*
  blood vessels and, 55
  CNS transmission and, 55
  cocaine abuse and, 66
  family of receptors, 54–55, 54*t*
  gastrointestinal (GI) tract and, 55
  metabolism of, 24
  methylenedioxymethamphetamine
    (MDMA) and, 54–56, 54*f*, 58
  nerve ending and, 55
  platlet aggregation and, 55
  receptors, transduction pathways effects,
    25*t*
  serotonergic neuron, schematic diagram,
    24*f*
  structures rich in, 54–55
Soldier's Disease, 3, 119
spice drugs, synthetic cannabinoids. *See
  also* marijuana
  CNS effect, 161–162
  mechanism of action, 161

peripheral effects, 161–162
  route of administration, 162
substance dependency, treatment
  behavioral therapies, 186–187
  chronic disorder, relapses to dependency
    and, 184–185
  cognitive behavioral therapy, 187
  combination therapies, 185
  detoxification programs, 185
  drug dependency factors, 183
  individual's neurological responses and,
    183
  Matrix Model, 187
  National Institute on Drug Abuse,
    effective treatment principles,
    184
  outpatient treatment, 186
  pharmacologic interventions, 186
  residential treatment, 185–186
  treatment effectiveness, 187
  treatment settings, 185
  12-Step Facilitation Therapy, 187

T
thebaine (paramorphine), 128
tolerance, defined, 9
treatment effectiveness, 187
treatment settings, 185
12-Step Facilitation Therapy, 187
tyrosine hydroxylase, 16–17, 17*f*

V
vin Mariani, 5
  addicts, 4

W
Wren, Christopher
  hypodermic needle, 3